# STEVEN J GOLEBIOWSKI

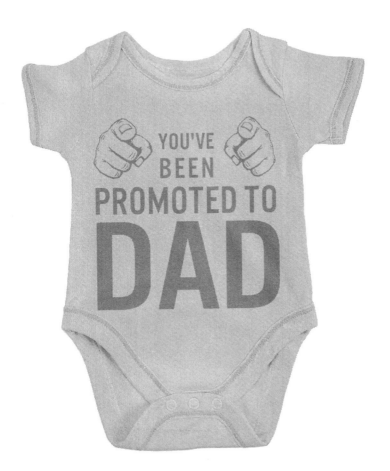

THOUGHTS, TRICKS, AND TIPS TO PREPARE YOU
FOR THE MOST IMPORTANT JOB OF YOUR LIFE

You've Been Promoted to Dad

Published 2017

Hermosa Beach, CA. 90254

www.promoted2dad.com

ISBN PAPERBACK: 978-0-9996549-0-3

ISBN eBOOK: 978-0-9996549-1-0

Edited By: Leslie Swaner

*This book is dedicated to the two loves of my life, Christian and Savannah. Thank you for promoting me to the best job I could ever dream of landing. I love you both infinity times infinity.*

# Contents

*Becoming a parent is permanent. Your child's youth is not.*

# FOREWORD

A little disclaimer before you read this book. I'm not a doctor, nor do I claim to be. I'm just a guy who happens to feel that my story can relate to most every guy (and maybe even a few women out there) who just got the bomb dropped on them that they're going to become parents. I hate reading, so the fact that I'm writing a book is a little strange to me. Over the course of my thirty-nine years on this planet, I could count on one hand how many books I've read cover to cover. Anytime I've ever read a book, I've always checked to see how long the chapters are, so out of respect to people like me that aren't big readers, I'll try and keep all the chapters in this book as direct and as short as possible. When my wife and I were going through our pregnancies, I read a plethora of chapters in a variety of pregnancy books that were all informative and educational. Most every pregnancy book out there does a good job of covering the medical procedures, the development of the fetus, and the changes happening to the woman's body. I couldn't, however, find a single book that really dug into the honest thoughts and emotions that the prospective father was going through.

In this book are my observations, my opinions, and my feelings during my wife's pregnancies. My memory can be challenged at times, probably due to all the brain cells I killed during college. As a result, I probably forgot to put a bunch of stuff in this book, but if I forgot to put it in here, it probably isn't that important anyway. I've organized this book in the simplest way I could: stuff that happens *before* baby is born, and stuff that happens *after* baby is born. I think it's important to talk about the first several months after baby is born because there are some things I learned along the way that might benefit "parents-to-be." I started writing this book soon after my son was born, and then finished it years later, after my daughter came into our family. There are times when I refer to my son in this book, and it might seem as though I don't acknowledge my daughter as I rehash some stories. It's not because I love my son more. I love both my kids equally. It's just that my son came into our lives first, so it was during my wife's pregnancy with him that I transitioned into parenthood and experienced many of these emotions for the first time.

A little bit about me... I come from a normal, middle-class family in the northern suburbs of Chicago.

I was a good high school athlete and hung with the "in crowd." I played college football at Indiana University, where I was also a member of the hardest partying fraternity on campus. I like to think we got all the hot girls. I used to chew tobacco, but I quit after my son was born because it isn't good for me. My favorite four things to do, other than being a parent, are: drinking booze, driving sports cars (really fast), snow skiing, and shooting guns. Oh, having sex with my wife is up there too, so I guess I'll bump up the list to my five favorite things to do, besides being a parent of course. Okay, I have to come clean about something. Although I did play football at Indiana, I never saw any real playing time. I blame it mostly on the fact that I was more interested in chasing tail and getting wasted than I was interested in studying my playbook. I'm telling you all of this not to beat my chest and tell you how cool I was (some, after all, might think this stuff makes me a dork), I'm telling you this because I want to paint a picture, revealing that I am a 'typical' beer-drinking dude, who loves sports and chasing beautiful women.

So, when I was presented with the idea of fatherhood, it scared the shit out of me! It scared the shit out of me not because I was worried I wouldn't be a great dad; instead, it scared the shit out of me because I was going to have to stop being selfish. I was going to have to start putting somebody else before myself. No more last-minute trips to the mountain when there's a fresh dumping of powder. No more drinking my lights out and sleeping it off the next day. No more having sex with my wife anytime or anywhere. No more relaxing on the couch and watching sports all day. For the first time in my life, I was going to have to answer to people other than myself, and those people were going to be my kids.

# BEFORE BABY IS BORN

# NATURE KNOWS WHAT IT'S DOING

It's where babies come from. The birds and the bees. The beautiful thing nature thought of called "sex." I have a little fascination with nature. When you look around at everything nature's done, it's pretty amazing. I'm not aware of any mistakes to date that nature has created. Everything nature has created has a place in this world. Even the bad things, like diseases, have their place; they serve a purpose. It's even more amazing that nature was smart enough to make the one act, vital to the procreation of life, so much fun!

It's obvious that nature would want sex to feel good because nature wants life to continue. Can you imagine if nature decided to have sex feel like a root canal? Nobody would be having babies. I know I sure as hell wouldn't be having sex if it felt like I was getting a tooth yanked out! I have sex because I love it, and it's the one thing that is always consistent. Sex, from the beginning of time, has felt good. I'm sure cavemen (and cavewomen) loved having sex, and I'm sure the people thousands of years from now, who live on Mars, are going to love having sex. When I watch Discovery

Channel, it looks like other species of animals like having sex too. Hell, my dog likes it so much he's willing to try it on a person's leg! So, with sex feeling so good, why is it that men are able and willing 24/7, but the women aren't? Why do girls need to be "in the mood"? I'm *always* in the mood! I could be dead asleep from working 24 hours straight, but if my wife tells me she's ready to go, I'll wake up at a moment's notice, splash a little water on my face… and it's on. But that isn't exactly the case for my wife. If she's sleeping, there's *no way* I'm getting her to put out, no matter how long I try to sexually arouse her. The reality is that guys are just hornier than girls. And I've never really understood why, until I started reading up on pregnancy and how the woman's body works.

Now, I'm not a scientist or a doctor, but if I understand the process of a woman's "cycle" correctly, a woman can really only reproduce a couple of days out of the month. No matter how good the "swimmers" are coming from the man, if the woman hasn't ovulated, she's not getting pregnant. It's that simple.

When I was younger and in high school, the sex education teachers scared the death out of us kids, making us believe that if we had intercourse with a girl, a baby was going to automatically come out nine months later. The reality is that's not true; there is a finite window of opportunity each month for the man's sperm to fertilize an egg. In fact, there are more days in each month when it's physically impossible for the woman's body to get pregnant. And I think that's by design. Nature designed it to be difficult for life to be created. The more difficult it is, the more it ensures that what life is created will be more apt to survive. I can't tell you how many friends I have that took months, or sometimes even years, to get pregnant. Very rarely do pregnancies happen in the first month of trying to make a baby. The window of opportunity to get pregnant is so specific, so precise, that most women can predict to the day when their best chances are of getting pregnant. There are even physical queues in the woman's body signaling that she's ready to reproduce. The woman's core body temperature changes, and her natural vaginal lubrication changes in consistency, getting more "sticky." Nature makes this happen so that our "swimmers" can have an effortless journey to meet up with the egg. Sort of like a Slip'N Slide for sperm.

However, I don't know why nature intended this, but us guys can reproduce everyday -- 24 hours a day. There is no downtime for us guys. Our balls can be called upon at a moment's notice, and every time we have sex, there's an equal opportunity for us to fertilize an egg. By that, I mean, our sperm is always capable of fertilizing an egg every time we release it. And I think that explains why guys have a ridiculously strong sex drive. Nature engraved in our DNA that we are fertile around the clock and, therefore, we should reproduce and reproduce often. The more we have sex, the better opportunity for the human race to survive. The reality is that if you lined up sixty women that were ovulating and had one man have sex with two of the women a day for thirty days, he could, in theory, have 60 women walking around with one of his kids. It's crazy to think like that, but it's true. The female body, on the other hand, just isn't built to reproduce like the male's. Reverse that situation: one girl has sex with 60 different guys over the course of 30 days. The reality? The female body can, at maximum, only carry a pregnancy by one man at any one time (although there are rare exceptions where paternal twins have different fathers). Point being, once she is pregnant, she will be pregnant and out of commission for any newcomers for the duration of her pregnancy. So, whoever fertilizes the egg first wins, and the other 59 guys have lost out on their opportunity to procreate with her. It's this fundamental difference between the male and female body that I feel explains the discrepancy in sex drive. Guys are always "ready to go" because nature has given us the ability to reproduce at any given second. But the girl is only "ready to go" *some* of the time because her body can only get pregnant *some* of the time. It's almost as if nature told the women, "what's the point in having sex if you can't get pregnant?" I'm guessing that maybe ten percent of the time my wife actually wants to have sex with me. The other ninety percent, she's just being a good wife and "taking one for the team."

# MARRIED LIFE

In today's world, you could probably say that my relationship with my wife before we got married was rather unconventional. My wife, God bless her, is from a traditional Hispanic family. So, her plan was to live at home until the day she got married. Let me tell you, trying to organize getting laid around a strict Hispanic mom isn't easy. It was hard work getting action in the early days of our relationship. Now, when most guys would love being able to have sex with a girl and then have her leave for the night, it kinda got on my nerves. The problem my wife and I ran into is that we could never *truly* relax. We couldn't pop a bottle of wine, cuddle on the couch, and then fall asleep. My wife would never drink more than a glass of wine because we both have a firm belief of *never* drinking and driving. Every night we hung out, prior to marriage, we always knew that we could never *really* get loose because my wife always had to drive back home to Mommy and Daddy's house. So, when we did finally get married, and she did finally move in, it was like "Hallelujah!" We were both so excited, we knocked back bottles of wine every night for the first I don't know how many months. Married life in the early going was great. We could finally relax, get buzzed together, make love, and fall asleep in each other's arms. Life was good.

I like to think we took advantage of the first several years of marriage. We traveled often, went to nice dinners, and genuinely had a good time together. In my mind, we did it right. We had a few years of fun as newlyweds, and then had the kids later. There's nothing wrong with having kids right away. In fact, now that I know how much I like being a father, if I had the choice, I probably would have bumped my fatherhood up a year or two. See, I really like being a dad, but it's not until you're a dad that you realize how cool it actually is. Being married and having fun as newlyweds was great but, for me, becoming a *real* family was when my life began to feel complete.

# I Don't Get Kids

Throughout my life, I never got kids. I never saw the cuteness in them. I never saw their innocence. I never understood why anybody would want to have one. To me, kids cried a lot and they were a pain in the ass. Before I became a father, I never felt comfortable with kids. Holding them was awkward to me. It didn't feel natural. I would try it from time to time by holding my brother's two kids. But even my brother's kids, my own niece and nephew, still didn't feel natural in my arms. There was something awkward about holding somebody else's kid.

# THE WEIRD THING ABOUT
# BECOMING A PARENT

The second my kid was born that "weirdness" of holding a baby disappeared. My son seemed to just "fit" in my arms. The second I held my son in my arms, for the first time in my life, it felt natural to hold a baby. It was almost like an old baseball mitt I had for a long time. When I put my son in my arms, it's like he belonged there. Looking back, prior to my son being born, holding babies made me nervous. I was this big football type guy, and I was afraid I was going to hurt *any* baby I held. The idea of supporting the head made me nervous; I was afraid if I moved a certain way, the baby could get hurt. Now being a father, I realize those fears are pretty ridiculous. I mean, yeah, you have to be careful, but holding a baby is really no big deal. Funny thing is, I saw that same fear and reluctance from my friends when *they* held *my* kids. I always liked to hand my son or daughter over to my buddies, and I saw how they would react. It was usually about two minutes later that they handed him or her back over to me. And when they held my kid, they didn't look good at it. There was that same awkwardness I felt before I became a father.

My friends held my kids like they were waiting for my kid's head to start spinning around. If you're a guy and you're reading this book, I can almost guarantee that you feel the same way I felt and all my buddies feel. But don't worry, when it comes to your own kid, he or she is going to fit like a good old pair of sneakers. But even today, although I'm comfortable with babies, I still have no desire to hold somebody else's kid. And the awkwardness comes back when I hold somebody else's baby. It sounds harsh, but even now, as a father, I really don't have the desire to hold anybody's kid but my own. I don't know why, but holding somebody else's baby just doesn't appeal to me.

# THE BLUE PLUS SIGN

I remember the day my wife told me that she was pregnant. What a day! We were married four years up to this point, and I wish I could say that I was jumping up and down excited when I saw that blue plus sign, but I wasn't. It had been more than 10 years since I was in college, but I still felt young and full of life. My body was in its thirties, but my spirit was saying I was still 19. I still had all kinds of things I wanted to do with my life, and I didn't want a kid slowing me down. I still had countries that I wanted to visit, and I wasn't anywhere close to where I wanted to be career-wise. The idea of a kid sounded limiting to me. I thought, "Maybe this kid is going to cramp my style," or "maybe I'm not going to be able to continue to follow my career ambitions." What's really effed up is that I was probably happier that my boys could swim than I was at the idea of becoming a father. The reality is that my wife and I were having unprotected sex for years leading up to that day, so a little part of me was starting to worry about my manhood. Maybe my joystick wasn't capable of producing a kid. When my wife came into the bed that morning to tell me she was pregnant, I could see the joy in her eyes, and I felt guilty that I didn't share her same excitement. I never led her to believe that I wasn't excited. On the outside, I gave the impression of joy. But on the inside, shit was hitting the fan. I could see my wife's heart pounding and she was glowing but, unfortunately, I didn't share that same enthusiasm. Instead of being excited to become a father, I was worried I would have to change my lifestyle. It's true what they say, a pregnant woman does glow during those nine months. I don't know if it's the extra blood in their body or what, but I read something in a pregnancy book that said a woman's body produces an extra two to three pounds of blood during those nine months. Or maybe it's just the fact that the mom is so happy because she is carrying and bonding with her child to be. Whatever the reason is, my wife was the most beautiful she's ever been during those nine months.

The first thing I did after my wife told me she was pregnant was go out to the local pharmacy and buy several different boxes of pregnancy tests. I was convinced that the digital one was the most accurate. By the way, that's a bunch of crap. I was surprised to find out that the digital pregnancy test isn't digital at all. The digital test is simply a housing that you put the regular pregnancy test into. Instead of you reading the line yourself, the digital one reads it for you. What idiot can't read a plus sign? Needless to say, I was disappointed by the digital pregnancy test; I felt like I got ripped off. To save the cash, I would almost recommend going to the *dollar store* and scoring a couple pregnancy tests there. For us, they worked just as good. The woman urinates on a strip of paper, and you get your answer just as quick as the $20 tests. Well, long story short, all the tests my wife urinated on turned up positive. My stomach was in knots. And if everything went as planned, I would be a father in less than nine months.

# The Big "M"

For any of you reading this book that don't want to visit any bad thoughts, I would suggest skipping this section. I believe in always staying positive during a pregnancy. I think being in the right frame of mind is good for both baby and mom. So, if you're feeling good and you've got some good mojo going, don't ruin it by reading something that could plant a bad seed. Just skip this section and get on to the happy thoughts. For those of you that want a little insight into the dreaded "M" word, my wife and I suffered two miscarriages before we had our son, and I'll do my best to share one of our stories with you.

I was in Connecticut on business when I got a call from my wife. She was crying, and I knew something wasn't good. Through the tears, she was eventually able to tell me that we lost the baby. It was a weird phone call for me. My wife could hardly speak she was crying so much. I had never heard her so upset. In fact, I don't know if I had ever seen or heard my wife cry up until that point. So, the fact that she was upset really bothered me. If I could, I would have reached through the phone and hugged her, but I couldn't.

Being hundreds of miles away, I felt helpless. I didn't really know what to say. I felt it best to listen. I tried to assure her that everything would be okay, but in that moment, nothing I could say was going to make her feel better.

One thing everybody can agree upon is that nobody ever wants to see somebody they love in pain. And my wife was in an incredible amount of pain, not so much physically, but emotionally. A few weeks before the miscarriage, my wife was two hearts beating as one. A space within my wife's womb was occupied by a life. Although small and primitive, it was still a life; it had a heartbeat. And then, in an instant, it was gone. The space that used to be occupied by our baby was now barren. I remember my wife telling me that she never felt so empty in her entire life after she suffered that miscarriage. As I listened and witnessed my wife's pain, I couldn't help but recognize the fact that I wasn't experiencing those same emotions. Even though my wife had experienced this intense feeling of loss, I didn't. In my mind, I figured we would just try again. It wasn't losing the baby that bothered me, it was witnessing my wife depressed. I hated seeing my wife sad, and I just wanted her to be happy again.

Because I wasn't having these same feelings of loss

that my wife was experiencing, I started to do some soul searching. I wondered why the miscarriage wasn't affecting me like it was affecting my wife. After all, I was the father of that baby. How come I'm not crying? I felt like I should have been more depressed. The more I thought about it, the more this idea of guilt started to creep into my head. I started feeling guilty that I didn't care more. I started questioning if I was a good father because good fathers would have cared more if their baby just passed away, right?

The only way I can explain the discrepancy of grief between my wife and me is that I never got to bond with the baby. Other than a pregnancy test saying that my wife was pregnant, life was business as usual for me. I had no evidence other than a blue plus sign that I was going to be a father. I never met the baby. I never touched the baby. I never saw the baby. I believe I didn't grieve because I was never given the opportunity to bond with that child. My wife, on the other hand, bonded with that baby the second the sperm met the egg, so it was logical she would feel the loss. Every day that she was pregnant, my wife would communicate to the baby in her mind, almost like praying. When my wife talked, she believed the baby was listening. I didn't have that dialogue with the baby. I never felt like it could hear me, so I never made an effort to communicate with him or her. For me, I didn't feel a need to grieve for someone that I had never met nor that I had ever loved.

I wish miscarriage wasn't a part of life, but it is. There are millions of couples that have gone through this, and there will be millions more. The "Miscarriage Club" I call it. It's a dark underground club that exists, but nobody really likes to talk about it... and for good reason. Who wants to talk about depressing stuff? The fortunate thing about miscarriages is they are not predictive of further miscarriages or permanent problems. Because a couple suffers one doesn't mean they are going to suffer another. And because a couple suffers two, like in our case, doesn't mean they are not capable of having children. Miscarriages are simply nature's way of saying something wasn't right. When the guy and girl's DNA starts to combine, something doesn't jive. And nature, being so ridiculously smart, decides to terminate the pregnancy. It makes sense that most miscarriages happen early on in the pregnancy because nature wants mom and dad to start trying again as quickly as possible. If nature waited later to terminate a pregnancy, it would have wasted several months that could have been utilized trying to reproduce. So many things have to go right for a baby to be born, it's a miracle that it happens in the first place. I never once during our two miscarriages thought for one second we weren't eventually going to find success. I put my trust in the process of life and found comfort in the idea that nature probably knows what it's doing. In my mind, it was just a matter of time before we could officially call ourselves parents.

# THIRD TIME'S A CHARM

So, after going through two losses, we were back to being happy. Nature had performed its little miracle, and my wife was pregnant again. The third time around was a bit different for me. This time I was genuinely excited. I didn't have those selfish thoughts of my life being stifled by a kid. I was a few years older, and possibly more mature. I felt like I was ready to be a father, so when my wife was pregnant the third time, I wanted nothing more than for my wife to have a successful birth. Looking back, I almost thought I jinxed the previous pregnancies. Maybe because I wasn't as "gung-ho" as I should have been, the pregnancies ended in miscarriage. I know that's ridiculous, but I couldn't help but wonder if my selfish attitude didn't contribute to our babies not making it. Maybe the babies got some weird intuition that I wasn't ready to be a father and decided it wasn't the right time.

One thing I can tell you about going through losses is that after you go through one, it's all you think about. There wasn't a day that passed during my wife's third *and* fourth pregnancies that I didn't think about losing my son or daughter. I know it was my job to stay positive, and I tried with all my might. I forced myself to think good thoughts, but there was always that little worry in the back of my head that something could go wrong. My wife and I never talked about it. But I think we both gave each other the impression we had no doubts, so the other wouldn't worry.

I remember one instance where my good friend Don got married. I believe my wife was a couple months pregnant at that time, but we hadn't told anybody. Seeing I was at my college buddy's wedding, I was pretty aggressive with drinking booze and I probably didn't realize how annoying I was being to my wife. I must have asked her three hundred times if she was feeling okay. As much as I was drinking and having a good time with my buddies that I hadn't seen in a long time, I couldn't stop from obsessing about my wife and if the baby was okay. Every thirty seconds, I would ask my wife, "Are you feeling okay?" Over the course of the night I was getting to my wife, and she finally snapped. She said, "YES! I'M FINE! STOP ASKING ME!" I think we ended up leaving the wedding shortly after that.

My paranoia continued until both my son and daughter were in my arms. Once my wife started feeling our son or daughter moving in her stomach,

I constantly asked her if she felt him or her. I think I was cool about it. I didn't ask her too often to let her think I was worried, but I knew if she felt the babies moving, then all was okay and he or she was still alive. As the weeks progressed, and we got closer to the end of each pregnancy, I can say my worries of losing them became less and less. As my wife's belly grew and I could see with my own eyes my son and daughter moving, my paranoia was ultimately replaced with excitement.

# Choosing the Vagina Doctor

It's always weirded me out… male vagina doctors. I think back to my college days and wonder what made that guy become a vagina doctor. Was he sitting with buddies drinking beer trying to figure out how he could look at women's private parts all day, and then it dawned on him, "I know, I'll become an OB! That way I can touch boobs and look at hoo-haws all day!" Fortunately for me, my wife had a female vagina doctor. So, I didn't have to deal with the insecurities of some man sticking his fingers in my wife's "area." Picking the OB is a big deal; he or she is going to be the one in charge when baby is being born, so you want to make sure they know what the hell they're doing. If you are planning on having a natural birth, you want to go over the doctor's history of C-Sections and drugs and make sure the doctor is okay with not intervening. I would suggest going to a couple different OBs and seeing which one both you *and* your partner feel most comfortable with. Remember, **your doctor works for you**, you don't work for them. You have the power to hire and fire whatever doctor you see fit to deliver *your* baby. If something about your doctor is rubbing you the wrong way, kick that doctor to the curb and find somebody else. Consider the location of the office when choosing a doctor. You're not going to want to drive an hour every few weeks to see the doctor. In the beginning of the pregnancy, the doctor visits are spread out, but when it gets closer to the big day, Mommy goes to the doctor more often. One thing some OBs don't tell you is that they are on call 24/7. So, if you have an appointment at two o'clock and another patient has just gone into labor, guess who wins? Sometimes you'll have to reschedule your appointment at the last minute, and if you drove over an hour to get there, it will probably frustrate you to say the least. So, I would definitely try and find a OB/GYN in close proximity to your house. The hospital is *another* really big thing to consider with regards to the doctor. Doctors are only allowed to deliver in certain hospitals, so if you had your heart set on a certain hospital, better make sure the doctor you are talking to can deliver there.

In Los Angeles, there are a lot of hospitals. I'd say there are fifteen hospitals within twenty miles of our house, so for us, we had a ton of choices when it came to hospitals. And if we had our way, we would have delivered at a hospital closer to home. But the doctor my wife chose only delivered in Beverly Hills so, based on that, we didn't have a choice but to deliver further from home. We weighed the pros and cons of switching doctors, but it didn't make sense to us.

At what point the doctor starts to intervene is a big factor for those wanting a natural birth. Intervention is when the hospital does *anything* that can interfere with a natural birth. An example of this would be giving Mom drugs to speed the labor process along (aka: Pitocin). My belief is that birth has become a business for doctors, hospitals, and drug companies. And like any business, the faster they crank through customers, the more they make. I don't believe a hospital would ever intentionally do anything to put Mom or baby's life in danger to make a few extra bucks, but they are in the business of speeding the process along a bit. It was important to my wife that her labor(s) progress as naturally as possible. She didn't want drugs to make her labor quicker or numb the pain. And she *definitely* wanted to avoid a C-Section. If going the more natural route is for you, check with the doctor to see if they are cool with taking a step back and letting the mom's body do what it's designed to do. Some doctors are cool with it, some aren't. In today's age, most doctors have warmed up to the idea of letting the labor progress naturally, but it's something to address if getting drugged isn't in your plans.

# MORE SPACE

Well, the family's growing, so it's time for more space, right? This is where I have a different point of view. Before we had our son, my wife and I lived in a small, two-bedroom house. Fast forward five years later, with two kids, and guess what? I live in the *same* two-bedroom house. I'm guessing our house isn't more than 750 square feet. It's two bedrooms with only a single bath. But you know what? We make it work. It's not ideal. It's not the most comfortable situation at times. But at the end of the day, it's our home, and we love it.

The first thing that both of our families said when we were pregnant with our son and then later pregnant with our daughter, was, "You better get a bigger house." And it wasn't like our parents were suggesting it, they were making us feel like we were being bad parents if we didn't. I thought about getting a bigger place but, honestly, I didn't want to spend the extra money. I was already going to be stressed becoming a new parent, why put the added stress on myself of having to pay for a bigger, more expensive house? And equally important to the money issue is I really like where I live. I'm a couple of blocks from the beach, and I live in a great neighborhood. Yeah, my house is going to be small for my kids, but they're going to grow up close to the beach. I want them to experience what living by the ocean is all about. I want us to be able to hop on our bikes as a family and pedal down the oceanfront boardwalk, stopping at cool oceanfront restaurants for lunch. I want my kids to play in the water on the weekends and bury me in the sand. I didn't *want* to leave.

So instead of giving into our parents demands, I held my ground and didn't look for a new house, but rather, I looked for ways to make our existing house work. Before my son came, I sold our living-room table and replaced it with a smaller one that I put in the kitchen. We had a monster fridge, so I sold that and replaced it with a smaller one, one that could fit in a more ideal place in the kitchen. I had a *ridiculously* huge couch that I sold and replaced with a more modest one. There are some really nice box storage units out there that help hide the toys. I bought a chest and put it behind one of the doors. It's amazing how much crap you can fit into a chest. In a matter of seconds, the house can go from disaster to clean with a big enough chest to throw everything in. But don't expect to find anything quickly if you decide to dig through it looking for something. Haphazardly throwing toys in a chest is a sure way to never be able to find a specific toy again. I've actually looked at the bottom of my chest to see if there was a trap door because as easy as it is to throw stuff in there, it's next to impossible to open it up and find a specific toy your kid is asking for. I can't even tell you how many times I've dug through that chest only to *never* find the toy that I know I put in there -- ever again.

Probably the biggest change we made when my son came around was switching bedrooms. I gave my son the bigger room. Logically it makes no sense to give the smallest human in the house the biggest room, but we did it anyway because although he was the smallest, he had the most crap. Cribs, rocking chairs, dressers... all that stuff takes up space. All said and done, we did what nobody thought was possible; we made a small, 750-square-foot house work with a baby. And then baby number two came along. And immediately we were pressured again: "Get a bigger house!" But, again, I had the same feelings I had when my son was coming into the world. I liked where I lived and I thought I could make it work. So to maximize our space, I started rearranging our rooms when my wife was pregnant with my daughter. My wife and I felt it would be better to *not* put my daughter in the same bedroom with my son because of all the waking and crying. So, we put my daughter's crib in our room. Still, I wanted to give my daughter the impression she had her own space, so I painted the corner of our bedroom pink, and decorated it as if she were in a completely different bedroom. I put up cute pictures on the wall and really tried to make the corner of our room feel like her own space. One of my absolute fondest memories of being a parent is having my son, who was two years old at the time, help my pregnant wife and I paint his sister's corner. My son wasn't talking very well at the time, but he could say a few words, and one of them was "WOW!" I put plastic all over the carpet, took my son's shirt off, handed him a paint roller, and he loved it! He was dunking that roller in the paint and spreading it all over the walls saying "Wow! Wow!" I knew giving my son that paint roller was going to get messy, I knew he was going to get paint all over himself, and I knew anything he painted, I was just going to have to go over and fix it. But you know what? I got the most brilliant beautiful video of my son painting his sister's walls. And anytime I watch that video, a smile spreads across my face from ear to ear.

Now, having my daughter sleep in our room was a *big* difference from my son sleeping in his own room from day one. The biggest difference in having a baby sleep in the same room as you, as opposed to a different room, is that you constantly hear them and, conversely, they constantly hear you. As my daughter grew, so did her relationship with her brother, and it wasn't long before we moved her crib into my son's room. I was shocked at how excited both of them were to be sleeping in the same room. I had shared a room with my brother up until he had gone off to college, and my wife had done the same thing with her sister, so for both my wife and I, having our kids share a room seemed natural because we both grew up doing it. But as my kids' little bodies grew, so did their need for bigger beds. So we, of course, went with bunkbeds. The day the bunkbeds were delivered might have been the single most exciting day in both my kids' lives. They could *not* stay away from them.

# THE WAIT

I think one of the hardest parts of the pregnancy was the waiting. It's like buying a new car and having to watch it sit in the driveway for nine months -- without driving it. *It's pure torture.* When my wife told me she was pregnant, I started getting antsy. I wanted to meet my baby... now! I didn't want to wait nine months. I remember getting a pregnancy app for my tablet. Within that app was a countdown. Every time I would open the application, it would show a picture of what my son, supposedly, looked like within the womb. I could page through the app and see just how many more weeks we had to wait. In the beginning, the end seemed so far out of reach. The thing I liked most about the app is that it showed the *actual* size of the baby. So, I would hold the tablet up to my wife's belly and we could see exactly how big baby was. The crazy thing? In the early weeks, baby is microscopic. And week by week, the baby sometimes doubles and even triples in size. It's no wonder Mom is always tired. It's because baby is hogging all the energy to his or herself.

During the waiting period, I remember buying a stethoscope. My wife and I were so excited to hear our baby's heartbeat, I thought if I bought a stethoscope I could hear it. Well, we used that thing a lot, and I never heard my son's heartbeat with it. I would probably recommend saving your money and not even bother buying one. I cheaped out and bought one online for around 15 bucks. The reviews were good, so I figured, "What have I got to lose?" My wife and I used the stethoscope often. And, the crazy thing is we heard a "swooshing" sound right out of the gate. My wife found it in the lower part of her stomach. We were pumped because we thought we found baby's heartbeat, but in actuality, we didn't. The "swooshing" sound was really my wife's blood flow *to* baby. Still, cool to hear, but not the heartbeat.

# DE-STRESSING

One of the things I wanted to make sure about while my wife was pregnant is that I didn't want her to *ever* feel stressed. I always wanted her mind to be at ease, and I never wanted her to worry. As corny as it sounds, I think baby picks up on Mom's feelings and emotions. I felt if my wife was stressed, it would in turn stress my unborn baby.

To help relax my wife, I went out and bought a nice docking station for the bedroom. The logic behind it, other than me getting a new toy, was to have my wife listen to relaxing, "spa- type" music before bed. I've always liked getting massages, and I've always liked how massage rooms feel very tranquil. So, I thought I would try and duplicate the spa setting in our bedroom. During the first trimester, I would turn off the lights and create a relaxing ambiance by turning on a few electric candles. My wife and I would zone out listening to relaxing spa music. It was nice in the beginning, and I actually looked forward to going to bed. I enjoyed getting a *real* chance to unwind. But like anything, if you do it long enough, it starts to annoy the shit out of you. It took about eight weeks before my wife and I were over listening to the spa music. And then, we went back to watching TV and going to bed like we had always done before.

# The First Doctor Visit

At about eight weeks is usually the first doctor visit. It's not a big deal, really. The doctor asks typical medical questions and draws blood to check different hormone levels in Mom's blood. Some doctors recommend an ultrasound this early in the game, but I personally don't think it's necessary, and I'll tell you why. Life is the most complex process on this planet. We humans think we have a grasp on it, but we don't. We currently have the ability to help start the process of life through different fertilization techniques, but once that process of life starts, there is nothing that modern medicine can really do to make sure that the pregnancy goes smoothly. From the moment of conception, it's solely up to nature to do its job, and all doctors can do is monitor the progress. So, at eight weeks, the baby is literally so tiny and fragile that I don't feel bombarding it with sound waves is really the right thing to do. Logic tells me that something that small getting disturbed by the sound waves that an ultrasound machine produces may actually cause harm, so why do it? I think the procedure is especially invasive because they do it by inserting an eight-inch ultrasound stick into the mother's vagina.

Early on in pregnancy, it's not done over the belly like in the movies. It's a pretty invasive process; one that I don't feel is really necessary that early in the pregnancy. However, there may be times when it is necessary, I just don't feel like it should be considered a "normal" part of the OB/GYN care process so, at the end of the day, do what you and partner are most comfortable with. I can understand the excitement of wanting to see the baby on week eight, both my wife and I wanted to see our baby too, but I also think it's a good opportunity to start practicing being a parent. By that I mean always putting your child's health and safety before your own wants and wishes. I think by rejecting the ultrasound in the early stages of pregnancy, you may be potentially protecting your child from sound waves that may or may not be harmful to the unborn child, no one knows. After our losses, when we found out my wife was pregnant with our son, we told our doctor we didn't want to do an ultrasound until later on in the pregnancy, and she was totally cool with it.

# So... Should We Tell People?

Once you find out that you're pregnant, I have to admit, it's exciting, so it's natural to want to share your news with family and friends. For our first pregnancy, my wife and I didn't waste any time. We called our parents and spread the news the second we found out; however, spreading the news early can come at a cost. If something should go wrong, and we learned the hard way, then you have to announce the bad news. The hardest call I had to make was telling my mom that we lost the baby. Emotionally and immediately, I accepted losing the baby. I accepted that he or she was gone and for all practical purposes, I had moved on within minutes. But I knew the news was going to be hard on my mom. My brother had suffered similar misfortunes, so I knew my mom was going to be crushed. When I told my mom that we lost our first baby, it wasn't good. My mom cried, which made me cry, and it was a pretty shitty situation all around. The second pregnancy, we kept our secret close to our hearts, for fear that if we did lose it, we didn't want our parents to be crushed again. It's a good thing we did because, just eight weeks in, we lost our second son or daughter. Not having to tell people kinda made it easier for me. I just kept our secret close to my chest, and nobody was the wiser of what we just went through.

Okay, no more depressing talk about losing babies. From here on out, it's only happy thoughts and positive outcomes. Now for our third and fourth pregnancies, they both went off without a hitch, and eight months after finding out we were pregnant, we had a beautiful boy and girl resting in our arms. For both my son and my daughter, we held off telling people until my wife reached the second trimester. They say if you reach the second trimester, then it's pretty much guaranteed that you're going to have your kid. So, the day my wife hit the second trimester in our third and fourth pregnancies, we called *everybody*. It was awesome to get it off our chests and share the news! We were so excited to be pregnant and, finally, we were able to share our excitement with everybody else. The beauty of waiting until the second trimester is that everybody can breathe a little easier. We weren't as worried and, in turn, our parents could relax a bit more. For us, waiting to share the news was purely circumstantial. If you feel like telling people, then stand on the highest mountain and shout it so everybody can hear, but if you feel like waiting, that's okay too. Take comfort in knowing that, statistically, your baby is going to be fine, and in nine months you'll be looking into his/her eyes for the first time.

# PICKING A NAME

When it came to picking the name, my wife and I were pretty bad about it for both my son and daughter. We browsed through various name books and scoured the Internet, but we never could find a name that felt right. We live in the Los Angeles area, so it's not uncommon for people around here to name their kid some unique name like, "Sky," "Apple," or "Blue Ivy". Because of all the unique names going around, my wife and I felt obligated to think of something outside of the box. We had a lot of weird names that were in the running for a while, and whenever we'd tell our traditional families, they'd roll their eyes a bit. I think it was so hard for us coming up with a name initially for my son because we didn't know his sex. We elected to keep it a surprise, so it was hard falling in love with a name because we didn't know what we were having. For my daughter, the name process wasn't as difficult because we elected to find out the sex during her pregnancy. But for my son, it became a bit of a fiasco.

The thing that is messed up about names is that when you hear a name, you tend to think of

somebody that you already know who has that name.
My wife would pick a name, and I would shoot it
down because I knew some guy in college with the
same name, and I hated him and didn't want my
kid growing up to be a prick like him. My mom
was always worried that when my kid was born, the
little card in the hospital bassinet would say "baby"
and not his or her *real* name. For my son's birth,
Grandma's worst fears ended up coming true because
my wife and I didn't pick my son's name until a few
minutes before we left the hospital. For almost two
days, my wife and I couldn't figure out a name. It's
not like we were arguing and my wife wanted one
particular name and I didn't. It's just that we never
could settle on a name that felt right. For my son, we
paged through baby name books, and nothing was
jumping out at us. When you get released from the
hospital, they make you fill out this form for the birth
records department, and on that form is the baby's
name. In our case, the birth records department was
closing in fifteen minutes, so we had to figure it out
fast. With the clock ticking, my wife and I were going
to have to settle on a name that my son was going to
be stuck with the rest of his life. I was firing through
baby name books, calling names out to my wife as

she held him and looked into our son's eyes. For us, the best way I can describe the "naming process" is that it kinda just came to us. I kept calling out names and, for whatever reason, I kept going back to "Christian". Never in the nine months prior to that day had the name "Christian" even been mentioned. But there we were, seconds from naming my child, and "Christian" kept popping into our heads. As I kept saying names out loud, my wife looked down at my son and felt he looked like "Christian." So, it was final. After nine months of not knowing what to name my son, in the final seconds of leaving the hospital, with the clock ticking, my wife and I made our first major decision as new parents. We would agree to forever call our son Christian James Golebiowski.

# SURPRISE OR NO SURPRISE

Prospective parents have to decide whether or not they are going to find out the sex of their baby. There are pros and cons for both. The big pro, obviously, is you can better prepare if you know the sex ahead of time. There aren't that many gender neutral options out there for newborns. I think with the advent of ultrasound, more parents are finding out than *not* finding out -- and the marketplace has adjusted to that. For my daughter, we found out the sex. For my son, we didn't find out the sex. Not knowing the sex for my son's birth offered a different set of challenges as opposed to finding out for my daughter.

The first obstacle in not finding out the sex is figuring out what color to paint the baby's room. If you know you're having a boy, it's pretty straight forward; your baby's room will probably have blue in it. If your baby is a girl, it's most likely going to have pink. But what if you don't know the sex of your baby? What color do you paint the room? What sheets do you pick? Not knowing the sex really limits the selection of bedding for the crib. So many bedroom sets are gender specific now that if you don't find out the sex, it can be really hard finding a bedroom set that you like. For my son, we ended up going with a green and yellow room and a bedroom set with the same colors. Now, I took my job of painting my son's room *very* seriously because my son was our first kid. I really wanted to make sure his room was perfect, so I went to the local paint store and I bought 15 different paint samples to put on the wall. I never knew how many shades of green there were in the world until I had to decide on one to paint my son's room with. I didn't want it too bright. I didn't want it too dark. Like *Goldilocks*, I wanted it "just right." I do recommend getting paint samples before you commit to a color because, in my experience, the color swatches in the store didn't quite match the color that ended up drying on my wall.

Now, if you don't find out the sex, along with having to keep the room gender neutral, you've got to keep the clothes gender neutral as well. You can't put a boy in a pink shirt and vise-versa. To me, most newborns don't look gender specific. What I mean by that is that I think it's really hard to determine a newborn's sex by just looking at the face, so the color of a newborn's clothes is sort of the way most people are able to distinguish whether your baby is a boy or a girl. It was a little difficult to find my son clothes before he was born because there isn't really *that* big of a gender-neutral selection. There are certainly more options out there for parents that already know the sex. But I don't really know if not having a large selection of newborn, gender-neutral clothes is really all that big of a deal. Because, the reality is, a newborn baby grows so rapidly that the newborn clothes don't really last you that long anyway. So, all you really need is about one month's worth of newborn clothes, and then you can shop to your heart's content once baby is here in the world and you know the sex.

Now the reality is that the room's color, the crib's bedroom set, and finding enough gender-neutral clothing options is really rather trivial. The one thing that I think is the most important thing to consider when deciding if you want to find out the baby's sex is your ability to bond with your unborn child. Having gone through a pregnancy both knowing and not knowing, I think I can offer some insight into the bonding process. Not knowing what the baby's sex is made it a little harder for me to bond with my son because I didn't really know if what I was talking to was a boy or a girl. I found myself talking to the baby and calling baby just that, "baby." I couldn't talk to baby like a son because I didn't know if my baby was, in fact, a boy. And I didn't want to talk to "baby" as a girl because I didn't know if she was, in fact, a girl. I had to always have general one-sided conversations with my son because I never really knew who (boy or girl?) I was talking to. I definitely think not knowing the sex affects the father's ability to bond. It certainly did for me. But then again, I don't know if my inability to truly bond with my son in the womb was a direct result of me not knowing his sex, or if it was just because I had never been a father yet. I can tell you when my wife was pregnant with my daughter, I had, at that point, bonded with my son on such a deep level that I think it was easier for me to bond with my daughter in the womb. During my wife's pregnancy with my daughter, I was already a parent and had fully made the transition from single dude to parenthood, so it was a completely different experience for me. I think, emotionally, I was more in tune with myself which, in turn, allowed me to be more in tune with my unborn daughter. I knew what it was like to love and be loved by a child, so I think I was at an emotional advantage for my wife's pregnancy with my daughter, and that made it easier for me to make a connection with her in the womb. And I wonder if I didn't know my daughter's sex during the pregnancy -- would my bonding process have been different with her? I still think, looking back, I don't know if I truly ever bonded with either my son or daughter while they were still in the womb. I loved them. But I don't think I ever truly bonded with them. It might go back to our miscarriages...I wonder if I had a defense mechanism kicking in that didn't allow me to truly fall in love with my children until I saw them, actually in this world, tangible and there for me to hold. I wonder if deep down, in the back of my brain, while I was constantly worrying about their health and safety during the pregnancies, if my mind wouldn't allow me to bond with them because I didn't know with one-hundred percent certainly if I was ever going to really get to meet them. Maybe our previous issues with our pregnancies affected me more than I realized.

With both my son and daughter, we didn't decide on a name until they were born. But I've had friends that knew the name of the baby *well* before they were born. I think knowing the sex, and thus being able to name the baby while it's still in the womb, might help with the bonding process. It was difficult for me to really talk to my babies because I wasn't addressing them by a specific name, and that may have affected the bonding process.

Having gone through both knowing and not knowing, I think I would recommend holding off on finding out the baby's sex, at least on the first one. I say that because imagine back to your childhood when Christmas, or whatever holiday you celebrate, mattered. I know I couldn't wait to open my presents. I had butterflies, sometimes for weeks, thinking about waking up Christmas morning and discovering what surprises lay under the tree. When you don't know the baby's sex, it's like waiting nine months for the biggest and best Christmas present you're ever going to open. You get butterflies wondering what surprise lay before you. For me, it was fun not knowing. I remember the first thing that crossed my mind the second my son was born. I immediately looked to see if it was a boy or girl. It was a really special moment, even though it lasted only a split second. My wife asked, "What is it?" and I announced, "It's a boy baby. He's a boy!" Me announcing to my wife that my son was a boy, *I own that moment*, not some doctor waving an ultrasound wand. Me, the boy's father, was the one who told my wife what she just pushed out into the world -- and *that* was a very special honor that I was lucky to have experienced!

# IS MOM REALLY GOING TO BE A BITCH?

I can't speak for everybody out there, but I can tell you my wife *didn't* turn into a fire-breathing bitch during the nine months of both *our* pregnancies. I'd heard all these horror stories of wives being "total bears" to live with but, honestly, mine wasn't. And I'm not just saying that because my wife will most likely be reading this book. I think the whole "moody" thing is rather exaggerated. Maybe personality traits are heightened during a pregnancy, so if a mom was difficult before she was pregnant, chances are she's probably going to be more difficult while she's carrying a baby. My wife has a very laid-back personality, and that didn't change. My wife did, *maybe*, ask me to do more things around the house when she was pregnant, but it didn't really bother me. I just wrote it off as being my job as the husband to pick up the slack a bit while my wife was carrying our unborn child. I can tell you that as the pregnancy progresses and the baby gets closer to full-term, the mom is absolutely going to be more uncomfortable physically. It really became a lot of added weight for my wife to be carrying around, and rather mundane tasks became difficult as the weight packed on and the baby grew. I think I saw my wife grow considerably more uncomfortable in the final weeks, but I never witnessed her complain about it. I think for her it was all just a part of being pregnant, so it never really got to her. My wife was always grateful to be pregnant, and that appreciation certainly affected her positive mood.

# Holy Crap, It Moved

Wow, what a day! The day the guy sees the baby move is pretty awesome. It's not all that different from the movie *Alien*. It kind of freaked me out a bit the first time I saw one of our babies move. We were just relaxing, watching TV before bed, when my wife said she kept feeling our son move. I paused the DVR and kept my eye on her belly. It didn't happen right away... I was staring at my wife's stomach for what felt like four or five minutes. Then, out of nowhere, a kick! It was the oddest and coolest thing I had ever seen. It literally looked like my son had punched my wife's stomach from the inside. It was awesome! And it was the first time I had witnessed concrete evidence that there was a life living inside my wife's body. Yeah, I had seen him on an ultrasound a few weeks earlier, but this was different. This was in the flesh. It was real. I wasn't witnessing a picture on a computer monitor that doesn't feel real; this was certifiable and witnessed by my own two eyes that a baby is alive inside my wife's belly. I can honestly say I got a little emotional. I immediately put my hand on my wife's stomach and waited for my son to kick again. He did! Now, not only did I see my son for the first time, but I felt him too! This weird excitement came over my body that was never there before, and I immediately asked my wife what it felt like. She couldn't really describe it -- and rightfully so. She said it kinda felt like feathers tickling her stomach. All I know is from that point on the connection started between my son and I. I could put my hand on my wife's belly, and I could feel my son, and he could feel me. If you're reading this and haven't gotten to that day yet, buckle up and enjoy the ride because when it happens, it'll be a rush.

# So Much Stuff

So, with the endless selection of baby products, what do you really need? I can tell you, in Africa, all babies need is a breast. So why we, in first-world countries, need *all* this stuff to take care of our kids is beyond me. My first bit of advice, if this is your first child, is wait and see what you get from friends and family. If you're lucky like us, and you're going to have a baby shower, you're going to get so much baby stuff you're not going to know what to do with it all. We had very generous friends and family that bought us more than we could have ever imagined. It can be exciting going into a baby store, and it's natural to want to buy things. But wait until after the baby shower because you are going to get so much stuff that it's really a waste to spend your own money on baby items if people are going to buy them for you anyway.

When you go to the baby store to register for items, it can be fun scanning products with that little wand, but only register for items you *actually* want and think you're going to use. Your friends and family are spending their hard-earned cash on you, so make sure it doesn't go to waste. It's weird to admit it but, even to this day, I love going to baby stores and looking around. There's something about baby stuff that is so cool to me. Before I was a dad, I would cringe at the thought of going to a baby store, but once you fall in love with a baby, it's hard not to like looking at baby stuff. Once your babies are all grown up, going into a baby store can almost be nostalgic.

One item I can tell you that you *have* to get is a baby car seat. I call it the "bucket". They won't let you leave the hospital unless you have one, so if you're planning on taking your kid home with you from the hospital, a bucket is a must. After that, it's all really personal preference as to what other products you buy. Usually the bucket comes with a stroller. I recommend *really* looking at the stroller and making sure it's easy to fold and light weight. Convenience is key here; you are going to be popping that thing up and closing it down, throwing it in your trunk on a regular basis, and you want to make sure it's functional and works easily for you. There are a ton of high end strollers on the market now, and I think a majority of them suck. They are way too bulky, and a lot of them make you take pieces off in order to break the stroller down. Really look at the functionality of the stroller, and don't buy one because some movie star is using it. Movie stars have personal assistants and nannies helping them deal with the impractical, trendy stroller they just bought. Us "regular folk" need to buy the most practical stroller out there that will help make *our* lives easier, not the one that is the most beautiful stroller on the market. Oh, and just so you know, you're going to buy like *five* strollers for your kids. I don't know why, but as parents, we all do it. It seems like I got a stroller for every day of the week. I have the stroller that the bucket clips into, then I have a light weight "umbrella stroller", and now with the birth of my daughter, I have a "double-wide" jogging stroller because I got the bright idea that I was going to take both my kids jogging with me every morning. As I write this sentence, my daughter is now two years old and my son is four. I've had the double-wide "jogger" stroller for about a year and a half... and I've never once gone jogging with it. But I *can* say, it does come in handy when we take the kids to Disneyland. It's a complete pain in the butt to fold and carry, but it's awesome to have a place both kids can sit when they get tired. The stroller is so massive you can't easily fold it and carry it in the seat with you when you drive on the Disney tram. I made this mistake several times, folding it and trying to cram it in the seat with me, while my wife and I juggled the kids. Then, a Disney employee pointed out that the last car of the tram has double wide doors where they allow families to put the strollers in the last car *without* having to break them down. Let me tell you... it's awesome having the ability to just role the stroller onto the tram and not have to worry about the hassle of having to break it down and carry it. In keeping with the theme of Disney, the other bummer about the double-wide stroller is it's a pain to bring on "Mickey's Train", so we usually end up parking the stroller at the train station, riding the train around the entire park, then getting off at the same place we got on. Because of the awkwardness of the stroller, we don't have the luxury of using "Mickey's Train" as a means of transportation to get us from one end of the park to the other.

As far as a crib, there is this concept of a "forever crib." Basically, it grows with your child; as your kid becomes a toddler, you replace the front of the crib with a toddler rail, and then when your child outgrows the toddler bed, the crib turns into a full-size bed with the use of the supplied bedrails.

Now all these options are extra. The toddler rail is extra as well as the bedrails. When we had my son, I bought everything on day one because I liked the idea of the bed growing with my child. But the reality is, life changes. And although it sounded good at the time, we never used the bed rails for my son because we ended up purchasing a bunk bed down the road. We did use the toddler rail for my son, but never used the toddler rail for my daughter. So, I guess every kid is different, and I would almost suggest waiting to purchase any kind of option that changes your baby's crib into a toddler bed or larger.

The other thing to consider when you're thinking about keeping your baby's crib for life is that it isn't always going to look like it did the day you bought it. Once baby starts teething, he or she will start biting anything in site, and the thing that gets the brunt of the biting is the crib. For my son, we ending up picking out a "Cadillac" crib. He was my first kid, so I wanted him having a bed "fit for a king." It was several thousand dollars and looked beautiful when we got it. But as soon as my son started teething, he chewed the shit out of that expensive-ass crib, and it ended up looking like it got beat with a weed-whipper. Because of the teething aspect, I absolutely recommend doing research on the crib manufacturer. Investigate where the crib is built, and make sure whatever stain or paint they are using isn't toxic. It's not something you really think about, but baby will bite that crib and most likely inadvertently swallow a bit of paint or stain, so you want to try and make sure it's made from the least toxic materials out there. Now most cribs comply to certain government safety testing, which should almost guarantee there is no lead in the paint, but there are some baby furniture manufacturers that take it to the next level and really try to ensure the stain they use is the least toxic on the market. The manufacturer of my son's crib actually posted the toxicity reports of the paint and stain they used on their website.

Aside from teeth marks, the other thing that will affect the look of the crib is belt buckles. Guys, just so you know, every time you wear a belt, and you bend down to pick up your kid, chances are good that the belt is going to scratch the shit out of the crib. So, guys, a trick to help keeping the crib looking better for a longer time is take your belt off before you pick up the kid.

Where baby sleeps when you bring them home from the hospital is usually something that will be debated. There are a lot of parents out there that have baby sleep in a bassinet next to their bed. My wife and I decided against the bassinet for both our kids. We, from day one, had our babies sleep in their crib. I didn't see the point in putting my kids in a bassinet only to have them have to learn to sleep in a crib once they out grew the bassinet. I felt like putting my kids in the crib from day one helped them understand the crib is for sleeping. And there wasn't any transition from bassinet to crib.

One thing you'll get taught to do in the hospital is to "swaddle" your baby. For those of you unfamiliar with a swaddle, it's when you wrap your kid up like a burrito. Some kids dig it, some don't. My son loved it. My daughter hated it. If your kid ends up being like my son, and really likes being swaddled, spend the few extra bucks and buy some swaddle blankets. Swaddle blankets are specially designed blankets that make the burrito wrapping process a bit easier. One thing you'll notice is that no matter how good you swaddle baby with a traditional blanket, he or she will most always figure out a way to wiggle one of their arms free. And once an arm gets free, it's over; the swaddle unravels like a ball of yarn. Specially designed swaddle blankets do a good job of pinning baby's arms down, so they can't wiggle free. The other nice feature of specially designed swaddle blankets is most have Velcro. The Velcro just helps speed up the process of swaddling by eliminating the tucking of the blanket. With Velcro, all you have to do is wrap and attach. Don't worry about bringing a swaddle blanket to the hospital. The hospital has tons of blankets, and the nurses will show you as many times as it takes for you to learn a traditional swaddle technique. I took the swaddling very seriously and really tried to perfect my method. No matter how precise I thought I was, my traditional swaddles never looked as good, or worked as good as the nurses'. My son always wiggled his arm free. But when the nurse swaddled him, he was snug as can be and never got his arms free.

Baby clothes are a little trickier. You want to have enough on hand, but if you buy too much, you risk never using it. I can tell you I witnessed my wife put *tons* of outfits in a bag for storage that still had the tags on them. It's almost like we didn't even have to do laundry for either of our kids. We probably could have just thrown out every outfit after they were done wearing it, treating them like they were disposable. Newborn babies grow so fast, it really is a waste to have a ton of outfits. For my wife and I, it was exciting to be having a baby, so we wanted to buy clothes for my son. When you see some of the cute outfits out there, you'll understand what I'm talking about. But my mom gave me the advice to not buy any because we were going to get a ton at the baby shower. She was right, we did get a ton of clothes, and I don't think we really had to buy any clothing for the first six months of either of our kids' lives. The reality is, there aren't that many different clothes manufacturers for babies. All the big baby stores carry the same brands, so in actuality, there isn't all that much of a selection. If you buy a cute outfit for your kid, chances are you'll probably receive the same outfit at your baby shower.

Burp cloths are a thing that I consider a necessity. My mom taught me a trick to use cloth diapers as burpee cloths. They are usually bigger than the standard burp cloths that you'll find in the stores, and you want the biggest area coverage imaginable to protect your clothing from your little one's spit-up. As a general rule, you can never have enough burp cloths on hand. I always got a little queasy watching babies spit-up before I was a parent, but having now lived through it twice, I can tell you, it's not a big deal. I describe spitting up kinda like a "vurp," others may call it a "sour burp." We've all had it happen to us, we eat a little bit too much at dinner and we belch, and well sometimes, that belch is a bit more then we bargained for as a bit of food comes up with the gas. That's what I think happens to babies when they spit-up. Their stomach isn't used to holding food yet, and they aren't exactly the best at telling us parents when they are full, so when they burp, a little bit of fluid comes up. It's not full-on stomach acid and bile, it's just a bit of formula or breastmilk that regurgitates back up the baby's esophagus. It doesn't have that horrible "vomit" smell, it really doesn't smell like much at all.

So, let's see, I've covered the bucket, stroller, crib, clothes, burp cloths, swaddle, what else is there? Really, the rest is just fluff. Oh, blankets, you are going to need a bunch of blankets because you always want to make sure your little one is warm. Yikes, you're going to need bottles too. I guess there is a bunch of stuff you're still going to need. With respect to our bottles, my wife and I went for the glass bottles because of all this talk about how bad BPA (Bisphenol-A, a chemical compound found in most plastics) is for you. I think most every plastic baby bottle out there is supposed to be BPA free, but I don't know if they really are, and we didn't want to take the risk. And since plastic is a direct derivative of fossil fuel, I try and stay away from as many plastic products as possible. The glass bottles worked great for us, but we did have a couple miscues and broke a few. Also, make sure you are using the right "number" nipple when you feed your baby. The size of the hole in the nipple is directly proportional to your baby's size and age. As the baby grows, so does the hole in the bottle's nipple. If you give a newborn anything but a newborn nipple, you are guaranteeing that the baby is going to choke and cough on the fluid because they won't know how to drink it as fast as the nipple puts out. As newborns get the hang of eating and eventually start eating more, the nipple hole size grows with them.

If your partner is planning on breastfeeding, then a pump really is nice, and I would almost go as far as saying it's a necessity. We froze a bunch of breast milk and had a ton on hand for those rainy days. It is a little weird opening the freezer for an ice cream knowing it's buried in your wife's breast milk. But you get used to it. As far as heating the milk up, a bottle warmer is something you can get. But to be honest, a stove with a pot of water works just as good, and takes about the same amount of time too. The thing I hate about the bottle warmer is cleaning it. There is going to be a few times when you spill milk inside the bottle warmer, for whatever reason, and there isn't really a great way to clean it. The bottle warmer manufacturer says you can turn it on with vinegar in it and the vinegar should help clean it, but then your house smells like vinegar for a little bit because it heats it up and vinegar steam permeates throughout the house. For my son, we used a bottle warmer, and for my daughter we just elected to use a pot with water to heat the bottles. It might tell you something, when as seasoned parents the second time around, we elected *not* to use the bottle warmer.

Since we're on the subject, when you're out and about, they make nursing covers for those moms who are breastfeeding. It's basically a cape that Mom wears while baby is feeding, so she's not flashing her boobs to the entire world. I know there are those people out there that think nursing is natural and it should be okay to flop their boobs out in public, but I think in today's world... it's weird. I'm a huge supporter of breast feeding; I think it's the best nutrition a baby can receive. However, I don't know if I believe a woman should necessarily bare her breasts in public. There have been times when I've seen mothers breastfeeding in public. I know it's natural, and I know I'm not supposed to want to look, but I can't help it. I always end up looking at the breast, it's a natural, *human* response. I think I'm pretty sly about it, and I don't stare at it, but the fact is, if there is a boob, I'm going to look at it. And I know every other guy in the world thinks that way too. We can't help it, we are drawn to boobs! Knowing that, I felt *way* more comfortable when my wife wore the nursing cover in public because then I knew other guys weren't looking at her boobs. Now let's talk about something a little less enthralling.

I would say one of the greatest products out there, in theory, is probably the shitty diaper trashcan. The idea of a garbage can that keeps the smell of poop out of your baby's room is genius... if it can be pulled off. But I can tell you, in my experience, they don't *exactly* work as planned. The smell doesn't disappear, it just gets trapped. And anything trapped needs to be freed eventually. The gross thing about the shitty diaper trash cans is they create one big log of disgusting soiled diapers. When you have to take the trash bag out to throw the diaper log out, you release a disgusting cloud of shit smell that has been trapped in that can for days. Imagine, those diapers have been marinating in that trash can for 48 hours. Then, all of a sudden, you release the fumes into the world. It's like getting kicked in the face by a mule! But, know that baby poop doesn't actually smell that bad in the early going. It's not until baby starts eating solid food that the diapers get pretty ripe. To combat the smell of the soiled diapers, I simply bought a normal trash can with a lid. I recommend getting one with a peddle, or one with an electric motion sensor so the lid opens automatically at the wave of the hand. Having to use a hand to lift the lid on a trash can put your baby in a brief moment of risk if your plan is to throw the diaper out as you are changing the baby. Baby's start to wiggle around, so if you have to use both hands to throw out the diaper, it leaves the baby at risk of falling. But having a trash can with a lid isn't enough to keep the bad smelling diapers at bay. If you throw poop-filled diapers in a normal trashcan with a lid, your kid's room is sure to smell like crap. A product my mom told me about are these mini plastic diaper bags, not all that different from the bags people use to pick up dog poop. The concept behind them is that you place the soiled diaper in the plastic bag, tie it up, and the stench stays confined within the mini-plastic bag. Then, you throw the mini-bag, with the shitty diaper in it, in the garbage can, thus rendering your trash can odorless. I found that this didn't exactly work perfectly either, but I think it's *way* better than the shit log produced by the shit diaper can, but there is still room for improvement. My wife and I experimented with how many mini-bags it takes to adequately conceal the stench. We found that on a real nasty diaper, three bags would usually do the trick. You're probably thinking that's a lot of bags, but we're not talking about a ton of money here. We bought our mini-diaper bags at Burlington Coat Factory. We used to be able to get them in a box of 100 for 99 cents, but the company must have wanted to increase their profit margin, so they started only putting 75 bags in the box for the same price of 99 cents. Even at 75 bags a box, you're still only talking about a fraction over a penny per bag. Over the entire time your kid is pooping in diapers, I'm guessing the bags only add maybe 30 bucks to your bottom line. Now, even with using the mini-diaper bags, there were still some nights when I would walk into my kid's room and it would smell like shit. Ideally, we would have emptied the diaper trash can every day but, in reality, we only emptied it when it was full. So sometimes, the shit smell would creep into the room.

Well, one day I was vacuuming in my son's room and an idea hit me. I learned a trick from my mom to sprinkle carpet deodorizer powder inside a vacuum's bag to help the bag from stinking. When you have a dog, and use a vacuum with a bag, every time you fire the vacuum up, it smells horrible. It helps to sprinkle carpet deodorizer in the vacuum bag to help mitigate that smell every time you turn on the vacuum. Going off this same theory, I decided to sprinkle some *Arm & Hammer* Pet Carpet Deodorizer in my son's trash can *every* time I put in a fresh plastic bag. Honestly, I think the *Arm & Hammer* helped. Ever since I started sprinkling a little carpet deodorizer in my son's trash can, we never really had another instance of my son's room smelling like soiled diapers.

So, to recap, I would recommend three things to keep the poopy diaper smell from overtaking your baby's bedroom. The first is a trash can with a lid, the second, is mini-diaper plastic bags, and the third step is to sprinkle *Arm & Hammer* Carpet Deodorizer in the baby's trash can. If you don't want to do any of these things, then I guess immediately throwing the soiled diaper in the trash outside would be the best remedy, and actually, that is *exactly* what we did for my daughter. I ended up buying a trash can with a lid and placed the can outside of our patio door, which was in close proximity to my daughter's crib, so every time my daughter went to the bathroom, we just threw the nasty diaper outside immediately, and the smell of soiled diaper never permeated the house. Okay, enough poop talk, now let's talk about baby monitors.

A monitor to keep an eye on your baby is nice to have. My parents didn't have a monitor, though, and I turned out just fine. But with the advent of technology, they make us believe we need to always have eyes on our babies while they're sleeping. I happen to be a paranoid parent, so I went with the monitor that has a movement sensor. Basically, there is a sensor you put under the mattress of the bed, and it detects movement from the baby. If the sensor stops detecting movement, then an alarm goes off. However, it can be kind of a pain in the butt to get the sensor working properly. You have to buy a piece of wood and put it over the springs on your baby's crib. This gives the sensor a nice flat surface to rest on. The monitor company doesn't exactly announce to the world that this additional step is needed. I just went to one of the big hardware stores and had them custom cut me a piece of wood. Once the sensor is working properly, you'll find that the first few days you're *constantly* staring at the monitor to make sure your kid is still breathing. I'm not sure if the sensor adds peace of mind or adds to the stress of parenting. I found myself waking in the middle of the night to see if the monitor was still picking up my son's breathing. In theory, if the alarm doesn't go off, you should be relaxed. But that wasn't the case with me because I started staring at that monitor's screen making sure the little pendulum was moving, indicating everything was fine. The other thing about the monitor with the movement sensor is that you have to constantly turn the movement sensor on and off. In the early goings, it's a real pain in the ass. Being new parents, you jump up at the sound of your baby crying, and thinking to turn off a sensor isn't always on your mind. I can't tell you how many times my wife and I picked up our son without first turning off the sensor. The second you pick up your baby, the sensor thinks baby stopped moving and alarms blare and scare the crap out of you *and* baby. My wife and I actually got into an argument in the early going because she wanted to stop using the sensor because we would always forget to turn it off, and the alarm would blare. Long story short, I refused to stop using the movement sensor, and my wife and I eventually got in the habit of turning the movement sensor off *before* we picked up our son.

The other thing about the movement sensor is that sometimes it goes off if your kid is sleeping at the far edge of the crib. The sensor lies under the middle of the mattress, and for the most part it does a great job picking up movement, but sometimes if baby has moved his or herself into the corner of the crib, the sensor doesn't recognize movement and the alarm starts blaring. Talk about scaring the crap out of you. Our alarm went off a couple times in the middle of the night, and I ran into that room so fast! Fortunately, anytime the alarm went off, it was a result of a false alarm, or us not turning the thing off. It's up for debate whether or not I would get the monitor with the sensor again. Part of me loves it, but another part of me thinks it just adds to my paranoia of being a concerned parent. I can tell you that I did not use the breathing monitor for my daughter. Oh, another thing about the movement monitor, at least with our model, the rechargeable battery was horrible and the video monitor would only last an hour or so before we had to put it back on the charger. It's a huge inconvenience if your charger is in the bedroom, and you are watching TV in the living room. I looked for an additional charging station to get around this problem, but they didn't sell them separately. So, I would find myself putting the monitor on the charger (in the bedroom) while I was watching TV in the living room, thus rendering the monitor useless because it wasn't near me to look at it. This is one of the reasons I loved the bouncy chairs and swings.

Swings and bouncy chairs are probably the only other two things I can think of. My kid *loved* his swing. It almost becomes a second baby sitter. You put your baby in that thing, crank it up and, for the most part, they're happy. My son took many naps in that swing, and I'd say it was money well spent. The swing is what allows you to get stuff done around the house. Put baby in there and your hands are free to wash dishes, do laundry, or whatever. But please make sure that the swing runs on both battery and A/C power. Some swings, believe it or not, only run on batteries, which is absolute insanity. My friend bought a swing that didn't allow it to be plugged into the wall, and he had a box, I shit you not, of at least a hundred "C" batteries. I could not believe how many batteries he had to buy for that baby swing. So just make sure you can plug the swing into the wall for power, or you'll be stuck spending hundreds on batteries. Now for as much as both my kids loved the swing, you'd think they would love the *vibrating* bouncy chair, but both my son and daughter *hated* it. We couldn't even get them buckled in before they would start crying. I think swings or bouncy chairs are individual to each baby. Some babies like the swing while some like the vibrating bouncy chair. You won't know until you give them both a try. Definitely put the swing on your shower list because they can be quite pricey. My wife's sister bought my kid his swing, so it saved us over $150 bucks.

The sheets and mattress for the crib is a given, but I will say this; your baby is going to be sleeping on that mattress for hours on end, so I would recommend buying a good one. Don't buy a cheap mattress and expect your kid to be comfortable. Sleep is one of the most important things for your child's health and for your own sanity, so spend the extra fifty or hundred bucks and get them a good one. Don't go cheap on the mattress! I squeeze tested every mattress in the store, trying to figure out which one felt the most comfortable to me. And usually, the mattresses with the higher price-tags felt better. For some reason, the cheap crib mattresses are hard as a rock, so it makes sense that a baby would be waking up constantly. It's because they are sleeping on the mattress equivalent of a piece of plywood. This is one item, that I would put in the "money is no object" category. Please spend the extra cash to make sure your kid is comfortable. And of course, after a good night's sleep, it's playtime for baby!

This means you're going to need some toys. But really, toys don't come into play until later on in your kid's life, and I'll touch on that a bit later. In the first few weeks, your kid really is just a blob that eats, sleeps, and poops. The real interaction doesn't come until later. Oh, and when that interaction starts happening, being a parent becomes *magical*.

# To Cut or Not to Cut

If any of you dads out there are doubting your ability to cut the cord, I can tell you, it's not a big deal. I was unsure I was going to be able to do it because I thought I would get queasy, but in that moment, there is so much adrenaline going through your body, cutting the cord becomes an honor. I wish I could say the scissors slice through the cord like a hot knife through butter, but they really don't. You kinda have to work at it to get the scissors to cut through the cord.

One thing I learned during the pregnancy process is the idea of *when* to cut the cord. I always thought you just cut the cord as soon as baby is out but, the more research I did, the more information I found about delaying the cutting of the cord. What I didn't know in the early going is that we, as parents, have the option to delay the cutting of the umbilical cord. Why would one want to delay the cutting of the umbilical cord you ask? Because the umbilical cord is where baby gets all its blood and nutrients from Mom. And there is a school of thought out there that thinks we should delay the cutting of the cord until it stops pulsating. The theory behind it is, when the cord is pulsating, it is still pumping fresh blood and nutrients into the baby's body from the Mom. If you cut the cord too early, you are robbing the baby of valuable blood that his or her little body needs. There have been studies done with regards to delaying the cutting of the cord, and most of them point to the fact that it's better for baby. My wife and I elected to delay the cutting, so my son and daughter could get all the blood from my wife that they deserved.

There is a new thing now where parents are given the option to save the cord blood. If you elect to bank your baby's cord blood, then you will not be able to delay the cutting. The blood that would have gone to the baby now is saved for a later date should you need it. The idea of cord blood banking didn't really sit right with me. I did my research and, ultimately, we elected not to bank it. The cord blood banks lead you to believe that you are, in essence, buying an insurance policy on your baby's life. But I don't think they are being completely forthright in their message to parents. See, from my understanding, stem cells are only good if they come from a perfectly healthy baby. So, if your baby gets a disease that could be treated with stem cells, chances are, the cells that were saved from their own cord blood have the same genetic defect that gave the baby the disease in the first place, thus rendering the stem cells useless. Where the stem cells become valuable is if your baby is perfectly healthy and someone else in your family gets sick. Then you can use your healthy baby's stem cells to help treat whatever condition *another* person in your family is fighting. I thought it was misleading on the part of the cord blood bank companies, and I thought they played into the fear new parents have with regards to their kid's life and they exploited that. My wife and I felt giving our son and daughter that blood was more valuable than saving it.

# CLASSES? REALLY?

My wife and I weren't one of those couples that ran out and went to a bunch of pregnancy classes. In fact, it wasn't until the third trimester of my wife's pregnancy with my son that we started talking about attending some classes. There are several options out there. My wife and I settled on a hypnosis-type class.

Full disclosure, I was a little leery of the whole "hypnosis" thing, but it was the class my wife decided upon, and I was going to support whatever classes she wanted to take. I figured, at the very least, I would come away with at least some information that would be helpful. I'm ashamed to say, the first thing I did when I got in the room was look around to see who had the hottest pregnant wife. I know, it's disgusting, but it's true. After I was done conducting my own pregnant beauty pageant, which I'm proud to say my wife took first prize, we started with the first hypnosis exercise. The teacher had us close our eyes as she put on some spa music. With our eyes closed, the teacher told us to imagine we were on a beach, and then we were supposed to imagine eating a lemon. Soon as we were told to bite into a lemon, I discreetly opened my eye to see how many people in the room were buying into this exercise. As I scanned the room, surprisingly, everybody was into it. After a little bit of time, the teacher had everybody open their eyes and then asked the room what had happened when we bit into the lemon. The first thought I had was, "what lemon?" Apparently, other people's mouths in the class started to water when she told them to bite into the lemon. It was supposedly a lesson in the power of the mind.

As the classes progressed, I saw my wife embrace the process, so I thought I might also. I tried to *really* participate in the hypnosis exercises, and at the end of every class, I often times found myself falling asleep. Now I don't know if it was a deep sleep, or if I was hypnotized, but I can say that I usually felt pretty good after I woke up. What was rather strange is that I don't think I was the only person to consistently fall asleep. I believe most of the class did as well. And like clockwork, when the teacher starts telling everybody to wake up, you somehow wakeup and return to consciousness. I do believe some part of my brain was listening to her as she talked to me in my sleep. So, if that was happening to me, I have to assume that the same thing was happening to my wife. Something must have been happening on a subconscious level that put my wife's mind at ease with the whole labor process because that is what the hypnosis classes are really about. It's really about putting the mom's mind at ease, embracing the idea that the woman's body knows what it's doing, and to just relax your way through the birth. After the fact, in talking with my wife, she really liked the hypnosis classes. She said it helped her visualize how her birth was going to take place. My wife kept going over in her head how she wanted the labor and delivery to go down. I don't know if it's coincidence or not, but my wife's birth experience happened *exactly* how she imagined it, for both my son and my daughter.

With the hypnosis class came a hypnosis CD. I thought it advantageous for my wife to listen to the CD before we went to bed so, every night, my wife and I would listen to the hypnosis lesson that would help my wife visualize a successful and stress-free birth. Now, I realize hypnosis classes aren't for everybody but, for us, I believe they worked. I walked into that class a skeptic and walked out a semi-believer. I say semi-believer because the class would like you to think that the woman can hypnotize herself into not feeling any pain. That might be the case for one out of a million, but for normal everyday girls, once active labor hits, anything they learned in any class goes right out the window. The primal instinct of motherhood kicks in, and the body just takes over and does what it needs to do to deliver the baby. I know there can be a lot of fear for first-time mothers about to give birth. Although I didn't go through it physically, I was completely present in the moment. And I believe it was the most beautiful and primal thing I've ever witnessed. The woman's body is one hundred percent designed to give birth. Take comfort in that. Nature designed the woman's body perfectly to be able to handle this.

# DOULA TIME A.K.A. THE BIRTH COACH

We live in Los Angeles, and us Angelinos tend to be a little strange when it comes to some things. One word I had never heard of until my wife got pregnant was "doula." I'm from the Midwest, so the way I grew up, the women gets pregnant, and she has the baby in a hospital... with a doctor. Well, now there are people called doulas.

Doulas are basically birth coaches. They can't deliver the baby, and are not licensed to do so. They are more of an "emotional guide" for the woman during the birth process. The idea of paying somebody to tell my wife when to push was a little ridiculous to me. Having this kid was going to cost me enough, why throw more fuel onto the fire? Well, my wife wanted a doula, so there was nothing that I could say to change her mind. Thus, we began the process of interviewing and picking the right doula for us.

We went to a "Doula Day" at a local birth clinic. The best way to describe Doula Day would be to compare it to five-minute speed dating. My wife and I were put in a room, then, various doulas would come in and we would talk to them. This is where I was introduced to some pretty effing weird people. I think you have to be a little "out there" to be a doula to begin with, so I wasn't *that* surprised when we interviewed a few. One doula we talked to was this old lady that said she had "special powers" to hypnotize the mother during labor. I checked out as soon as she said she had special powers. Are you fucking kidding me, special powers? Who the fuck did she think she was, *Superman*? Then there was this African American lady that both my wife and I actually really liked. She was sweet and had a great personality. But I couldn't get over her voice. When she talked, she had this soft sweet voice, and then, mid-sentence, it would change into a deep man's voice that really creeped me out. When she left the room, my wife and I talked about how we both really liked her. But then I brought up the elephant in the room. I asked my wife what she thought about her voice and my wife started laughing. My wife didn't think I noticed it. I said, "Of course I noticed it, who the hell wouldn't?" She went from female to male in a split second. I thought it would be distracting to my wife during labor when this sweet African American lady, all of the sudden, turned into a man *right* when my wife was supposed to be pushing. Long story short, we didn't find our doula when we went to Doula Day, so the search continued.

With Doula Day being a bust, I got on the computer and searched for a doula in the area where we live. Sure enough, a few popped up. I ended up calling one on the phone, and she seemed pretty cool. My wife and I scheduled a meeting, and we hit it off well. Problem was, she already had two women that were due around the same time as my wife, so she couldn't take us on as clients. So great, we finally find a doula with a normal voice, that doesn't think she's *Superman*, and we can't hire her. The doula was bummed she couldn't be there for us too, but she did give us a recommendation for another doula named Jenny. We met with Jenny and something just clicked. I liked her. My wife liked her. So, we immediately hired her to be with us during my wife's birthing day.

I must say, the nice thing about having a doula is the peace of mind. If you've never gone through the birthing process before, it's nice to have somebody in your corner, other than the doctor, that has witnessed multiple births before. If my doula was calm, it made me calm. For first-time parents, there are a lot of unknowns with regards to the birthing day, and it can be quite scary at times, for both the mom and dad. I didn't know what to expect when my wife went into labor. The only knowledge of labor I had was what I saw on TV, and I can promise you, it doesn't happen like it happens in the movies. In real life, it takes hours for the woman's body to prepare to give birth. So, the doula was crucial in educating my wife and I about the actual process of labor. We had a lot of questions for the doula, many revolving around what to expect. What are we to expect when the water breaks? How will we know it's time to go to the hospital? What can we expect once we get to the hospital? What's the difference between early, active and transitional labor? These were all questions the doula was able to answer for us. Our doula was also crucial in helping us to write our birth plan.

"Birth Plan" is another term I had never heard of until my wife was pregnant. For those of you not familiar with a birth plan, it's basically your "wish list" of how you want your birth to go. Couples write up this birth plan, usually a page long, and you give it to the hospital when you arrive. This ensures the nurses and doctors all know what your wishes are with regards to natural birth, C-section, drugs, etc. I'll talk more about the birth plan a little later. But I think it's crucial if you are planning a natural birth.

In addition to answering questions and helping us

with the birth plan, our doula was great at helping us ask the hospital staff the right questions. When you are caught up in the moment of labor, the hospital has a tendency to take over. Instead of asking you what you *want* to do, they usually will *tell* you what to do. Having a good doula in the room will help ensure the hospital doesn't push you in a direction you don't really want to head down.

# The Birth Plan

Think of a birth plan as a wish list. If the parents could close their eyes and dream up the perfect birth, that's what is supposed to be written on the sheet of paper. For parents that want a natural birth, your birth plan should stipulate that. If Mom doesn't want to feel any pain, then you put in the birth plan that you want the epidural. It's nice to give the hospital staff a general idea of how you envision the birth process to take place, so they can adjust accordingly. Not every mom is alike. Some want it natural, some don't, and it's impossible for the staff to know your wishes unless you write it down for them. It's important that the birth plan is short; try and keep it to one page. Change the margins if you have to. You don't want to be handing the hospital staff a 200-page dissertation on your ideal birth because they won't read it. It's probably best to use a format similar to an outline because that way the hospital staff can scan it over quickly and pick up on the major points. I was extremely happy with how the nursing staff immediately read the birth plan when I handed it to them. They did their absolute best to honor and respect my wife's wishes. There was one intern that I felt was maybe trying too hard and didn't really have anything to do. Because as my wife was laboring, she was relaxed in her own little zone, when this young doctor showed up, asking her questions about her pain level, which is rated on a scale of 1 to 10. I was briefly infuriated he asked those questions because I *clearly* stated on the birth plan *not* to reference any pain or hurt. Before my wife could answer, I cut her off and looked that doctor right in the eye and asked him if he read our birth plan. He said, "No". I told him not to come back in the room until he had read the birth plan. He never ended up coming back in the room, which leads me to believe he never read our plan.

I've provided a copy of our birth plan to give you an idea what ours looked like and, as you can see, it really sets the tone for the delivery. On the very top of our birth plan it is clear that my wife wanted this process to proceed as naturally as possible. Our birth plan was broken down into four sections. First Stage of Labor, Second Stage of Labor, Third Stage of Labor, and Baby.

In the *First Stage of Labor*, we made it clear that my wife wanted a calm and peaceful setting. She didn't want to be confined to the bed, she wanted freedom to walk around, and she didn't want anybody offering her drugs for pain or to speed the process along. In the *Second Stage*, where labor gets really intense, we asked for more of the same. My wife wanted freedom to walk around the room to try and get the baby out naturally. There are tools the doctor can use to help pull baby out of Mom. They can use a suction device, which is literally just like using a vacuum. A hose, not all that different from a vacuum hose on your home vacuum, is attached to baby's head allowing the doctor to pull baby through the vaginal canal. My wife and I wanted to absolutely avoid this if we could. There is nothing natural about that, and when you look online at some of the pictures of the babies' heads after the suction device is used, it borders on insanity. Another tool doctors can use are forceps. They are basically like large BBQ tongs. The doctor clasps the tongs on baby's head and pulls baby out. That didn't feel very natural for my wife and I either, so we *clearly* stated on our birth plan that we wanted to avoid assisted delivery. We also made it clear we wanted limited *assisted* delivery, such as using any suction device or forceps to remove the baby, only as a last option.

At the end of the second stage of labor, your baby is born, so on the birth plan is a map of instructions on how we wanted those first minutes to be conducted. We wanted our son and daughter to be *immediately* put on my wife's chest to allow bonding and breastfeeding. We wanted to delay the cutting of the umbilical cord until it stopped pulsating, and we delayed the eye ointment for one hour to allow maximum bonding between baby and my wife.

The *Third Stage of labor* is basically when the mom gives birth to the placenta. We wanted the placenta to come out as naturally as possible, so we clearly said no drugs to induce the placenta delivery.

# THE GOLEBIOWSKI FAMILY BIRTH PLAN

*GOAL IS TO ALLOW LABOR TO TAKE ITS NATURAL COURSE, FREE OF DRUGS and ANY UNNECESSARY INTERVENTIONS or REFERENCES TO "*MOVING THINGS ALONG*"*

## FIRST STAGE LABOR:

- **Hypnobirthing:** Please refrain from references to "Pain" or "Hurt". Respectfully decline discussion of pain tolerance and pain levels.

- **Calm and Peaceful Setting:** Dim Lights, Quiet, Soft Voices, Music.

- **Monitoring:** *Intermittent* using Fetoscope and/or Doppler.

- **Pain Relief Options:** Please do not offer, only if Mom asks. Would prefer *Relaxation, Positioning, Shower Accessibility, Heat/Cold Therapy, Massage, Acupressure.*

- **Mobility:** Respectfully ask for the freedom to walk and move around.

- **Induction:** *Only Natural Forms.* Walking and Nipple Stimulation.

- **Augmentation:** No Augmentation via Pitocin or Amniotomy.

- **Video/Pictures:** Father and Doula free to takes pictures and videotape.

- **Saline Lock:** No use of Heparin.

**SECOND STAGE:**

- **Positions:** Ask for the freedom to choose positions for the encouragement of baby to come down.

- **Spontaneous Bearing Down:** Ask staff to remain calm with low tones and gentle encouragement, free of "pushing" prompts, allowing mother to listen to body, while using Hypnobirthing breathing down techniques until crowning takes place.

- **Squat/Birthing Bar:** Ask that a squat/birthing bar be made accessible.

- **Episiotomy:** _NO Episiotomy_. Would like to use Massage, Oil and Hot Compresses, and/or Positioning to avoid this procedure.

- **Assisted Delivery:** Avoid the use of suction and/or forceps if at all possible.


**FOR BABY:**

- **Immediately Following Delivery:** Ask that Baby be immediately placed on Mother's chest allowing time to bond, while using mother's body heat to warm baby. Please refrain from using bright lights.

- **Cord Cutting/Clamping:** Delay clamping or cutting until cord stops pulsating. We ask that the _FATHER_ cut the cord.

- **Breast Feeding:** Breast feeding only.

- **Separation:** Baby is to always remain with parents and never to be taken out of room.

- **Eye Ointment:** Delayed one hour allowing time for Baby to bond with parents.

- **Hepatitis B:** _NO_ Hepatitis B shot

- **Vitamin K:** _YES_


THIRD STAGE:

- **Placental Delivery:** _Natural Placental Delivery_ using Uterine massage and/or nipple stimulation to assist with birth. **No** Cord Traction, Pitocin, or manual removal.

# To Have Sex or Not to Have Sex... That is the Question

Well, it's the same thing that got you into the situation you're in right now. So, when your partner gets pregnant, is having sex off limits for the next nine months? Sorta depends on the situation. Our doctor *and* all the books I read say that sex during pregnancy is perfectly okay. In fact, some books say that the woman's hormones are so sky high during pregnancy that some get horny as rabbits. I didn't have that problem. My wife's sex drive was about the same as before she got pregnant. But having gone through a couple losses, both my wife and I were a little scared of going at it all hot and heavy. We didn't want to do anything that might jeopardize the baby's wellbeing. If you're scared to have sex during pregnancy, I think it's perfectly natural. One technique we used early on was we would play "Just the Tip". The guy doesn't need to jam his penis in all the way to get off. A guy can just put in a quarter of it to get the job done. My wife and I waited for four months before we played "Just the Tip". Another thing you can do is get creative with it. My wife actually brought home a weird masturbation device that was made of this jelly material. The front of this thing was in the shape of a mouth, so it wasn't the most pleasant thing to look at. But what it lacked in looks, it made up for it in feel. My wife and I were nervous to have sex because we were both so protective of our baby, so we improvised and played around with different toys that allowed us to be intimate without putting stress on ourselves, and fearing we were hurting the baby. It goes back to the "not being selfish anymore." A couple years ago, I wouldn't let anything get in the way of me having sex. But now that I was thinking about my son or daughter, I was able to sequester my sex drive a bit because it was more important to me that I didn't do anything that would risk another miscarriage. I absolutely know that none of our two prior miscarriages had anything to do with us having sex, but a little part of me was nervous about having aggressive sex while my wife was in the early stages of pregnancy.

Talking to some women, I've heard a lot of them say they had body image issues as their bodies got bigger through the course of the pregnancy. For some women, they think pregnancy makes them fat and unattractive. For me, I found my wife to be the most beautiful she had ever been while she was pregnant. The bigger my wife got, the sexier she was to me. It goes back to that whole "glow" factor. Women glow when they are pregnant, and there's nothing sexier than a woman carrying your child. My wife carried herself with a certain energy that was intoxicating. I genuinely saw that my wife was happy to be pregnant, and it made me happy seeing that. I guess what made her even more sexy to me is that I knew that the baby in her belly was mine. I did that to her. As sick, twisted, and male chauvinistic as it sounds, it's almost like an ultimate mark of territory. By me getting my wife pregnant, I announced to the world that she was my woman. I did that to her and weirdly, it turned me on that she was carrying my child.

# HAVING SEX TO START LABOR

For those couples that are scared to have sex during the first eight months of pregnancy, there is light at the end of the tunnel. From what I've been told, a baby is considered full-term at around 38 or 39 weeks. That's when the baby's lungs are developed and can, in theory, be born and be perfectly healthy. It's not always the case, but I guess it's a general rule. Once that magic 38th week hit for my wife and I, it was game on. Our holistic doctor encouraged us to have sex and said it would help my wife into labor. Supposedly, there is something in semen called *prostaglandins* and they help soften the cervix. Not sure if prostaglandins are enzymes or hormones, don't really care either, I just know prostaglandins was my green-light to start having sex again… aggressively. See, the cervix is this big muscle keeping the baby inside Mom. When a woman has contractions, the body is actually opening the cervix, so the baby can come out. When the doctor talks about how many centimeters the woman has dilated, what they are referring to is how big the opening of the cervix is getting to allow baby to pass out of Mom.

So, when 38 weeks hit, my wife and I were like

rabbits, having sex any chance we could get. I swear, we made up for the 38 weeks prior. Morning, noon, and night, it was every guy's dream situation. It didn't matter if my wife was in the mood or not, she still wanted to have sex because she wanted to meet our kid. I wish she wanted to make love to me because she was horny and I turn her on day and night, but the reality is she wanted to have sex with me to meet our baby. Whatever the reason, I was happy to be having sex again on a consistent basis. I have to tell you, having sex with a 38-week pregnant woman is not the easiest thing to do with a basketball on Mom's belly. Missionary is pretty much out of the question. Doggy style isn't all that comfortable for the women either because they have a thirty-pound weight hanging off their body. Our position of choice was when my wife would lay on her side. It has the right angle where I could do my thing and it was comfortable for my wife. She could relax with her belly being supported by the bed. I wasn't really that well versed in that position prior to my wife being pregnant, but I can say that now after experimenting with it during the pregnancy, it's become one of my go to moves.

# HORMONE LEVELS

I don't really know anything about the different hormone levels in the female body. And I'm not qualified to start writing about them. Talk to your doctor or read another book. All I know is that there is talk that progesterone plays a role in a healthy pregnancy. Because we suffered a few losses, we monitored my wife's hormones like hawks in the early going of my son's pregnancy. We saw a dip in progesterone levels that made us nervous, so my wife's doctor put her on progesterone. It was basically a suppository that my wife put in her vagina that, in theory, would raise her progesterone levels. I don't know if it helped or not, but in the early stages of our pregnancy with my son, it did give us a little peace of mind that we were doing something that could maybe help our chances at a healthy pregnancy.

# Gestational Diabetes

A test Mom is going to have to go through is the blood glucose test. Doctors want to make sure the mother's body is breaking down sugar efficiently. Doctors test this by having Mom drink an orange soda and test her blood sugar level after she drinks the liquid. If the mom's sugar levels are high, it means she has gestational diabetes. Basically, the mom is diabetic during the pregnancy. Getting gestational diabetes isn't the end of the world, I know, because my wife had it for both of our pregnancies.

When the test came back that my wife was positive for gestational diabetes, she was pretty bummed. I think because it scared her. She didn't really know what that would mean to the health of our children. That golden ticket of my wife getting to eat anything she wanted during the pregnancy got thrown out the window. We had to meet with a nutritionist at the hospital, and my wife was put on a very strict diet. In its simplest form, my wife had to limit the amount of carbo-hydrates at every meal. She didn't cut out carbohydrates, she just limited them. It's important for women with gestational diabetes to watch their sugar intake because too much sugar for the baby is bad -- just like too much sugar for us adults is bad. If a mom has diabetes and doesn't watch her sugar intake, the baby can literally grow too big by becoming too fat in the mom's belly. So, it's really important that the mom monitor what she eats so she's not giving her baby too much sugar and making them unhealthy in the womb.

I didn't want my wife to worry about what she ate, so I took the worry away from her. Every day, I got up and made my wife's entire food for the day. I cooked her breakfast, lunch, dinner, and snacks. I followed the nutritional guidelines the hospital gave us, and it took the guesswork and worry away from my wife. Because we followed the hospital recommendations verbatim, my wife was able to keep her blood sugar under control and didn't have to go on any drugs to control her blood sugar. Just like any diet, moderation is key. Every now and then, if my wife got a craving for ice cream, she'd indulge. She just couldn't indulge *every day*. What's crazy about gestational diabetes is it literally up and vanishes like a fart in the wind once the baby is born. Within hours of both my son and daughter's births, my wife's diabetes was gone. What we did come to find out though is that women who get gestational diabetes are ten times more likely to get diabetes later on in life. So, even though the diabetes is gone after the birth, it's still a good idea for Mom to watch her sugar intake the rest of her life. But sometimes, that's easier said than done.

## Baby, If You Ain't Drinkin', I Ain't Drinkin'

It's obvious a woman shouldn't drink alcohol during pregnancy. But what about the man? I started thinking about it, and felt a little guilty having a beer or a glass of wine, knowing my wife couldn't partake. So, being the standup guy that I am, I made a pledge to my wife. As a show of my solidarity to her, I told my wife I wouldn't drink for the nine months she was pregnant. If she couldn't drink, then neither would I. Well, my pledge of sobriety lasted all of about three days. Okay, let me make clear that I'm not a heavy drinker, but I do like to enjoy a beer or glass of wine every now and then, especially if I had a rough day at work. So, giving up the booze really wouldn't have been *that* big of a deal for me. I was totally committed to it. What messed the whole plan up was that I realized that if I stopped drinking, I would be throwing away one of the best opportunities of my life. I would be throwing away the gift of having a designated driver for nine months. It was like having a taxi cab on duty all day, every day. What man in his right mind would squander that gift? Well, down the hatch the booze went, and my wife, being the saint that she is, was totally cool with it. She gave be a pardon on my pledge and drove my drunk ass around every now and then. I asked my wife on several occasions if she ever craved wine or beer during pregnancy, and her answer was always the same: she had zero desire to drink while she was pregnant. I think for her, she was able to shut it off instantly, for the simple reason that she didn't want to hurt the baby. It all reverts back to selfishness. Once you become a parent, you don't have the luxury of being selfish.

# Time to Get Fit

When the man finds out he is going to be a dad, there's this sudden moment of clarity. We all walk over to the mirror, look at ourselves and think, "fuck I'm fat." I was once a collegiate athlete, and in my prime I was a stallion. Fast forward twelve years later, I was a plump piece of shit. For the last ten years I had stopped working out, but didn't think to eat less, so it caught up to me. I was probably 30 pounds overweight, not a big deal, but enough for me to want to do something about it. So, then came the pledge to get fit while my wife was pregnant. It was going to be perfect. I had a clearly defined goal. By the time my son was going to be born, I would be 30 pounds lighter. I had nine months to do it, it was going to be easy.

Long story short, I didn't lose a single pound through my wife's pregnancy. It's not that I didn't want to do it, I did. I just simply couldn't find the motivation I needed to get my lazy ass into the gym. It kinda reverts back to the fact that a guy isn't a father until the baby is born. We think that when our partner gets pregnant, it will motivate us into getting healthy, but it doesn't. It doesn't because the guy doesn't know what they are in for yet. If they knew at the second of conception how amazing it is to be a father, then I think getting in shape would be a little easier for the guy during pregnancy. For me, the *real* motivation to get healthier didn't come until *after* my kids were born. As I started getting older, I started thinking about all the things I might miss out on if I didn't get my shit together. Slowly, over time, I gradually adjusted my lifestyle to include better choices. I'm not perfect, but I do absolutely feel the motivation I carry in my heart to be there for my kids as they grow up has helped motivate me to become healthier.

The problem with working out when you have a family is that it's a catch-22. With a busy work schedule, and without a lot of free time, you are constantly confronted with the questions: Should I go work out? Or should I go rush home to see my kids before they go to bed? It's not an easy question to answer; both have their advantages and disadvantages. Half of me wants to work out so I can stay healthy for my kids, and the other half feels guilty for not spending that time with my kids. I try to make it work by balancing it. I don't work out every day. I go when I can, and I always try to spend any free time with my kids. I can tell you that I didn't lose a single pound during my wife's pregnancies, but since my son and daughter have been born, I'd say I'm down 20 pounds.

# PACKING THE HOSPITAL BAG

One of the things you'll need is an overnight bag for the hospital. It's not a big deal, really. For the dad, think about it as… you're going away for the weekend. What would you bring? I packed a few changes of clothes and some toiletries. I would recommend shorts and a few comfortable t-shirts. The room is going to be very warm because it's important that baby be in a warm environment, so having shorts and t-shirts will help deal with the warm recovery room.

Other than the clothes, I'd say the next big thing for Dad to pack is a good camera. Make sure the camera battery is fully charged and there is plenty of storage on the memory card. It's a good idea to get a camera that is easy to use because chances are Dad will be busy helping Mom push out a baby, so somebody else in the room will have to take pictures. I made the mistake of bringing a complicated DSLR camera, and most of my pictures suffered as a result. The focus was way off, and I ended up with a ton of bad pictures because the camera wasn't user-friendly. A really good point-and-shoot camera is the way I think is best for hospital pictures because things will be happening at a fast pace once active labor starts, so you aren't going to have time to set up pretty shots anyway.

Setting the mood, I think, is another big part of the hospital bag. I wanted to try and promote an environment of relaxation, so I brought a nice wireless Bluetooth speaker and had spa-type music albums playing in the background for my wife. I also brought a few flameless battery candles to help set the mood. If you have time, and most of you will, you can turn down the lights, turn on soft music, and help Mom try and relax through the contractions.

Entertainment for the dad and mom could become important if you are being induced because you'll be in the hospital for several hours before baby comes. *I-pads* with a selection of movies and/or books seems to be the thing to do now. Just make sure you bring the charger for any electronics you bring with you, *including* your cell phone. Last thing you want happening is to have your cell phone battery die, just as your baby comes and you want to call all your relatives.

The last thing for dad would probably be his wallet. Make sure you have some credit cards *and* some cash because you are probably going to leave the hospital at some point and you'll need some money to get your car out of the parking garage. They charge for everything at the hospital, and parking is no exception.

As far as the woman's bag, I went all out and put all kinds of stuff in there for my wife. The first obvious thing you need to pack is an outfit for baby to go home in. You won't put baby in this outfit until you are just about to walk out the door. The next thing I would recommend is a soft blanket for baby. You most likely are going to want to shield baby from any elements when you are walking from the hospital to the car. Our neighbor's grandmother knitted us a really great blanket that we used to bring both my kids home in. Other than the stuff for baby, my wife packed a couple robes, slippers, comfy clothes and her toiletries. I packed all this extra crap they recommended like lip balm, lollipops, and granola bars but we never touched any of it.

## PICTURE ME ROLLIN'

One thing that the dad has to make sure is ready for when Mom goes into labor is the car. I backed my car into the driveway, so when it was go time, all I had to do is hit the gas and I was on my way. I didn't want to have to bother backing out of my driveway. If Mom is in active labor, time is money, and you want to make sure you don't waste valuable seconds. Dad, obviously, also needs to make sure there is enough gas in the car. I don't think my wife would have liked it if I had to pull over at a gas station on our way to the hospital. It can get messy in the car. The reality is, if Mom is in active labor and her water has broken, as was the case with my son's birth, there is probably going to be leaking fluid and blood. I'm a pretty anal guy when it comes to my car, so I bought a couple packages of doggy-poopy pads and taped them all over the seat and floor of my car. They are basically huge flat diapers for people that are too lazy to walk their dogs. The whole idea of doggy pads is a little strange to me. I can't understand why somebody would rather have the dog piss and shit in the corner of the house, as opposed to walking the dog outside, but that's an entirely different book.

The most important thing that has to happen with respect to the car, and is essential to the baby's well-being, is the <u>proper installation of the car seat</u>. It's not exactly rocket science. Parents can call the fire department, or drop by your local station to make sure the seat is installed properly. I didn't elect to call the fire department because I think I had a pretty good handle on it. The only real thing you have to remember is to make sure that bad boy is in there tight and it doesn't move. I am a bit obsessive-compulsive when it comes to my kid's safety, and installing the car seat was the first manifestation of that. I probably spent four hours putting my son's car seat in my truck for the first time. I tried it on the passenger side. I tried it on the driver side. I tried it in the middle of the seat. I tried it with a seat protector under the seat. I tried it without a seat protector under the seat. I tried it using the latch restraint system. I tried it using the standard seatbelt. After trying the setup 20 different ways, I settled on using the latch restraints, and I put the seat in the center of the back seat. Putting baby in the center of the car made it seem safer to me. I thought, if I ever got into an accident where I got hit in the side of the car, having my son furthest away from the door might be safer. I'm not 100% sure that is the case, but logic and common sense brought me to that conclusion. Now that I have a daughter I, of course, have seats on both sides of the car. A trick I learned when installing the baby seat 20 different times is apply pressure by leaning down on the seat. Basically, put all your body weight down on the baby seat so that you compress the car's seat cushion. This will allow you to get the strap at least an inch tighter. A tighter strap means a safer seat. Never should you be able to grab baby's seat and move it side to side across the seat. It needs to be anchored securely into place like a rock.

# THE BIRTHING DAY

So, the "Big Day" is just that... a *very* big day! It's a big day for Dad, but an even bigger day for Mom and baby. If Mom is planning a natural birth, like my wife did the first go around, she is going to have to go through something she's never experienced before. And, my personal opinion, is that it's the father's job to support Mom in *any way humanly possible*. My wife made up in her mind that she was having a natural birth, and I'm proud to say that she did it. My wife, all 110 pounds of her, pushed something the size of a watermelon out of a hole the size of a lemon. It was the most impressive thing I have *ever* witnessed in my life, and I am forever proud of my wife for doing it. My wife will tell you that she thinks the meditation classes worked great for her, and they really helped in the early stages of labor. But once active labor hit, everything was thrown out the window. Active labor is intense and it gets your heart going. Guys will never know what it's like to experience the right of passage the mother goes through in giving birth.

Child birth is a slow process, with labor happening for several hours. From what my wife tells me, the first part of labor is not a big deal. She kinda checked out and relaxed through the contractions. As a matter of fact, my wife started having contractions at 11 p.m., and she was nice enough to let me sleep the entire night. It wasn't until six a.m. the next morning, when I woke up, did she tell me she thought she was in labor.

From beginning to end, my wife was in labor about 15 hours. It sounds like a lot of time, but a majority of it wasn't a big deal. Granted, I was just an observer of the process but, from what I observed, my wife didn't mind the early labor stages at all. When my wife felt a contraction come on, she just relaxed through it. Giving birth is nothing like the movies. Labor doesn't happen like the flip of a switch, and all of a sudden you have to rush to the hospital. Labor is a very slow, gradual process that builds over time. Now, I'm sure there are certain exceptions to the rule, but for the most part, labor is a long process. It takes time for the woman's body to open up enough to allow the baby to pass through. The mom doesn't "all of a sudden" start screaming and you have to rush to the hospital. Labor is a very slow and gradual process. I think what helped my wife through the contractions is that she embraced them. In my wife's mind, every contraction meant she was one step closer to meeting our son or daughter. She was comfortable with the process and put her trust in the fact that nature knew what it was doing. My wife wasn't going to have to tell her body what to do. Her body was naturally going to do what nature intended it to do. My wife labored in the comfort of our home until the shit hit the fan. But when the shit hit the fan, boy did it ever. Because my wife wanted to labor at home, it was kinda up to me to assess the situation and decide when we were going to leave for the hospital. Leaving too early and my wife wouldn't be happy laboring in the hospital; leaving too late meant danger to the baby and possibly having baby being delivered in the car. I get asked a lot about how I knew it was the right time to leave for the hospital, and my only answer is "you'll know." There is a switch that flips in active labor. The woman almost checks out because she's going through so much pain. There's something primal about it. I could tell my wife's contractions were so strong she couldn't even handle them anymore. Her body was literally trembling through the pain. I witnessed nature taking over. My wife no longer had control of her body; my wife's body now controlled her. Once I saw this change, I knew we were getting close. Then, during a contraction, my wife's water broke. It was a little messy and there was blood. I wasn't alarmed by the blood because our doula said we would most likely be seeing some because the body has a tendency to bleed as it is opening up. Once I deemed it imminent that we leave, I helped my wife to the car, and I floored it to the hospital.

The drive to the hospital was one of my favorite parts of the experience. For the first time in my life, I was able to drive like I always wanted to. I viewed my wife's labor as a ticket to drive as fast as humanly possible. I drove like a bat-out-of-hell... speeding, running red-lights. I did what needed to get done to get my wife and son to the hospital as fast and as safely as possible. I was actually trying to get pulled over. I thought if I got pulled over, I could get a police escort. My wife, during the entire ride, was in active labor, which means she was screaming a lot. I wish I could say it was the same wonderful screaming I hear when I'm having sex with her, but it was nowhere close. She was screaming like I never heard her scream before. You'll notice that people are pretty cool with you if they know your wife is in labor. I would pull up to a red light in the left turn lane, roll down the window, tell the driver my wife was in labor, and everybody was really cool. I got a ton of "congratulations and good luck" from people. Once we arrived to the hospital, I pulled up to the emergency room and the nurse wheeled my wife up to our birthing room. They hooked her up to a heart monitor, gave her an IV for fluids, and oxygen.

I can say that it *did* get a bit stressful for me once we were in the hospital. You can't help but fixate on the baby's heartbeat once Mom is hooked up to the monitor. For whatever reason, my son's heart rate would fluctuate, depending on my wife's position in the bed. The doctors were keeping a close eye on the baby's heartbeat and, without giving us any indication they were concerned, would casually encourage my wife to move positions to see how that affected the baby's heartbeat.

After about an hour of laboring in the hospital, my wife was ready to push. I do remember, in that split second, when the doctor said that my wife was ready to push that time stood still for a beat. I literally remember thinking to myself, "This is it. This is a defining moment in my life. A crossroads. I came to the hospital a boy, and I'm going to leave a man. After nine months of waiting, the moment to meet my baby has finally arrived."

I got next to the hospital bed and grabbed my wife's legs; I held them back and encouraged her to push and breath. I just followed the doctor's lead and showered my wife with nothing but positive thoughts and encouragement. The awesome thing is I had a bird's-eye view of my son being delivered, and I can remember it clear as day what it was like to see his head for the first time. The first vision I ever had of my son was seeing a head covered in jet black hair. The crazy thing about watching a delivery is that a newborn's head is so soft that it can squish together during the delivery. As my wife pushed my son out, his head wrinkled and looked like a walnut as it squeezed out of the vaginal canal. Once his head was out, I told my wife. I watched our doctor clean out his airways and nose with a suction tube. Once Doctor felt my son's airways were clear, she asked my wife for a few more pushes, and he was welcomed into the world. Remember, we didn't know the sex of our baby up until that point, so I was looking to see what we were having. Once I saw my son's polish sausage, I yelled out, "It's a boy!"

The beautiful thing about nature is during the labor process, the female's body releases hormones, and one of the purposes of one of the hormones is amnesia. Nature is smart enough to release a hormone so immediately after the child is born, the mother literally forgets the pain she just went through, so she can bond with her new baby.

The second my son was born, he was on my wife's chest, and they were looking into each other's eyes for the first time. My wife encouraged my son to latch on, and he instinctively found my wife's breast. While he was on my wife's chest, the nurses cleaned and wiped my son down. I cut the cord, and that was it. My son was in our lives forever. I gave my wife a good 20 to 30 minutes with him before I held him. I thought it best that baby and Mom get those first precious moments together. I got a little emotional seeing my son laying on my wife's chest. I leaned over and kissed both of them. It was a pretty surreal moment.

After my son and wife had their time to bond, it was time for the usual stuff. The nurses took my son to measure and weight him. At this point, the hospital will usually put ointment on baby's eyes and give them a couple shots. A Vitamin K shot and a Hepatitis B shot. We elected to have the eye ointment put on my son's eyes. But we delayed it, so he had the first hour to look at us. I didn't want my kid's eyes covered in goop when he was trying to see Mom and me for the first time. The other thing we allowed the doctors to do was to give our son the Vitamin K shot. I'm not really sure if it was necessary, but I figured… it was Vitamin K, so it wasn't that risky. They give it to babies because it's supposed to help their blood clot. Although we went with the Vitamin K and the eye ointment, we elected *not* to give my son the Hepatitis shot. I thought it was a bit much to give my son a vaccine the second he was welcomed into the world. I wanted to give his body a little rest instead of blasting it with a virus the second he was born. When you really look at how people get Hepatitis B, I just didn't feel like there was much risk of my son being exposed to it at such a young age, so we elected not to give it to him.

After watching my wife and son bond a bit and getting the medical stuff out of the way, it was time for me to hold my son for the first time. To be honest, I kinda expected the clouds to part and angelic music to start playing, but it didn't. As a matter of fact, it was quite the opposite for me. When the doctor handed me my son for the first time, I remember looking down into his eyes and literally saying, "Nice to meet you, I'm your daddy." I kissed him on his little head, and I told him I loved him. I didn't have this warm fuzzy feeling all over my body. You know, the one you expect to feel from watching movies. Holding my son for the first time was almost like meeting a long lost relative. I knew I loved my son in that moment because it was the right thing to do, but because I really didn't know him yet, I didn't have that unbreakable bond that I was expecting from the second I laid eyes on him. I think it's attributed to the fact that I was never a dad up until that moment, so I didn't really know how to feel or how to act. The only analogy I can think of is to look back on a time when you started a new job. Were you great at that job on the first day? Probably not. You had to learn how to do that job over the course of a few weeks. So, I think that's why my love for my son started off smaller than I expected and grew over time. It's because I had never been a dad before, therefore I had to learn, over time, how to love him properly. Feeling those warm fuzzy feelings wasn't going to come naturally, it would be something I would have to learn *and* earn over time.

Every day since my son's birth, my love for him has grown exponentially. I didn't have those fuzzy feelings on day one, but I can tell you this: I have them now. There isn't a day or hour that goes by that I don't think about my son or daughter. And the second I do, a smile instinctively comes across my face. Often, I will page through pictures of my kids on my phone and, without fail, every single time I look at my kids' pictures, a smile creeps across my face. I don't tell my face to smile, it just does. It's almost become a joke at work. My co-workers always know when I've been looking at pictures of my kids because I have this "proud daddy" expression on my face that people can spot a mile away.

I don't really know if I just did a good job explaining what I felt the day my son was born because, to be honest, it's rather hard to explain. I think I just want all the dads out there to know that it's okay if you don't have a warm fuzzy feeling on day one. Don't think something is wrong with you, or that you're not going to be a good dad. I think it's rather natural for first time dads to be a little emotionally numb on day one because it's all so new. The bond and love one has with a child grows day-by-day, it doesn't happen all at once. And it won't be long before seeing your kid will become sorta like a drug. You will *literally* need to see them and hear their voices every day in order for your life to feel complete.

# AFTER BABY IS BORN

## Baby's Here, Now What?

So, an hour or so after baby is born, they put everybody in a post-partum room. Both my kids were born in Beverly Hills, so our rooms were pretty nice. I can say that the first nights with both my son and daughter... I never wanted them to end. The rush of the births was over, my adrenaline was gone, and I had this Zen-like feeling throughout my entire body. For my son's birth it was particularly special. I just can't describe what it was like to finally have him in the world with us. After suffering two losses and then making it through nine months of quiet worrying, I could finally take a breath. I could look down into that plastic bin and see my son breathing. I remember my wife and I stayed up most the night talking about what we just went through. We smiled, we laughed, and there was this overwhelming sense of relief. It was a great moment my wife and I had together, being parents for the first time. It's a conversation I will *never* forget.

When you get in the post-partum room, be prepared for it to be hot. As soon as I walked in the room, I asked the nurse to turn on the air conditioning, but it was here that I got my first lesson since my son's birth in not being selfish. The hospital intentionally set the room temperature high, so my son could stay nice and warm. For big guys like me, that room was sweltering hot. But to my son, it was as cozy as the womb he just exited. I'd say it took me about an hour before I got used to the warmth and then I didn't even think about it. We were assigned two nurses. They came in every so often, checking on my wife and son. Our nurses were really good about showing us new parents how to swaddle and change my son's tiny diapers. It made the transition into parenthood much easier. I got a real sense that our hospital was used to working with first time parents; they were very patient with us and welcomed any questions we had with open arms.

Immediately following the births of my son and daughter, my wife wasn't exactly ready to be doing any jumping jacks, so the responsibility fell on me to take care of my son and daughter for the first few hours of their lives. This was the magic time for me. I had been waiting nine long months to meet these little people, and now I finally got to prove myself to them. I changed all but maybe two diapers during our entire stay in the hospital. While tending to my children and changing their diapers, I experienced one of the most joyous things a dad will witness: The Meconium dumps.

Meconium is the first *real* poop your kid will ever take. When my son unloaded, he kept unloading. Diaper after diaper I kept putting under his little butt, and he kept filling the thing up. It's the strangest looking poop. It looks like and has the exact consistency of hot fudge. Seeing that Meconium is just another sign that baby is doing well.

After my son and daughter took their first poops in the real world, it was time for their first baths. It's no big deal really. Basically, until the umbilical cord falls off, you just wipe baby down with wet towels. The hospital staff gave my son and daughter their sponge baths as I just watched.

The umbilical cord was something I wasn't quite ready for as I became a new parent. See, when I look down at my stomach, I just see a belly button, but the belly button doesn't appear until a few weeks after baby is born. For those first few weeks of life, babies have a long chunk of umbilical cord hanging from their stomach. The hospital douses the umbilical cord in this blue liquid that is supposed to dry the cord up until it eventually falls off on its own. When it does dry up, it ends up looking like a piece of beef jerky. As a matter of fact, a friend of mine's dog ate their baby's umbilical cord after it fell off on the floor. Pretty gross if you ask me.

Since my wife breastfed our kids, there was a lactation consultant that came to our room to help teach my wife how to get my son and daughter to latch on to her boob properly. Believe it or not, some babies need help with it. And even though my wife became very good at it as the months progressed with my son, she needed a refresher course when my daughter came along. One thing I'm a little reluctant to tell you is that my lactation nurse for my son was pretty darn sexy, so it was a little weird watching a sexy nurse squeeze my wife's breasts. Part of me wanted to get turned on, but I think the dad reflex kicked in, and it didn't allow me to get aroused.

# WE'RE COMING HOME

Taking both my son and daughter home were *very* special days, but I must admit, taking my son home was particularly special because he was my first kid. The day I took my son home was day one of a chapter in my existence on this earth that started to complete me. As I write this chapter of the book, I'm looking at a picture of my son. He is only a day and half old in this picture. I'd just buckled him into his baby car seat, and he's looking at me through the back window of my truck. He is dressed in all yellow with the cozy knit blanket draped over him that my neighbor's grandmother handmade for him. I slid open the back window and jumped into the bed of my truck so I could get the right angle for the perfect head-on picture of him. As I look at this picture, I notice a look on his face. He wasn't scared. He wasn't nervous. He was curious. He was curious, wondering what all this was. It was the first time he had ever seen a truck before. It was the first time he had ever seen the outside. It was the first time he had ever smelled fresh air. This day marked the first day of my fatherhood in the real world, and marked the first day of my son's journey through life.

I loved driving home with my son in the backseat. I felt so at peace. I felt so relaxed. It just felt right. It felt like something I was destined to do. I don't know why some people are chosen to be parents and some aren't. I don't know why my son came into my life at the time he did. Maybe it was because I was ready for that transition into the next chapter in my life. I was sort of in a stalemate with my job, and I was unemployed, struggling to transition into a job that would be more fulfilling. I put so much pressure on myself to become this successful movie and television producer that, over time, I began to wear blinders. I was so focused on where I wanted to be career-wise that I couldn't stop and enjoy anything. I felt that if I wasn't a successful producer, I almost didn't have a right to have fun. My career was *everything* to me, and in examining it, I was a failure. Because I wasn't as successful as I wanted to be, it made it hard for me to *want* to be a father. I wanted my career set before I had any kids because to me they seemed like a distraction. I assumed that if I had a child, I wouldn't be able to put the necessary focus on my career. And if I couldn't focus 100% on my career, I was afraid I wouldn't become successful.

So, there I was, my career was in the toilet, my wife and I were scraping pennies to stay afloat, and I was driving home from the hospital with my son in the backseat. Logic would tell you that a situation of having a family and no income to support them would lend itself to stress but, for me, it was the complete opposite. For the first time in a long time, I felt like everything was going to work out just fine. I didn't care that I wasn't where I wanted to be career-wise, something in my heart told me that "bigger and better things" were around the corner and that I shouldn't worry so much about them. This whole time leading up to being a father, I thought fatherhood would be a burden, but it was the exact opposite. It was freeing. I finally started seeing the world again -- without blinders. I stopped being so obsessed about my career and started to obsess about something that really mattered. I started obsessing about my son, and then later, that obsession would migrate to my daughter as well. I started obsessing about being the best father I could be. It dawned on me that the most important job in my life had *nothing* to do with movies or television shows. The most important job that I will *ever* have is giving both my kids a safe, loving environment where they can be free to be who they want to be without fear of judgment from me or my wife. We live in a pretty fucked-up world when you really think about how people have tendency to judge one another. Kids in grade school can be real pricks, and now with the advent of social media, you get bullied in front of the world.

I'm ashamed to admit it, but I was once a bully. I think it was because I was bullied when I was younger because I had exceptionally large ears. So, when I got bigger, I thought it necessary to return the favor. Having lived on both sides of the coin, I'm pretty confident both my son and daughter are in for the same judgment. Growing up, I was that "asshole kid" that treated other kids that weren't like me as inferior. If I could go back in time and take back all the bad stuff I did to other kids, I would. Because it's not until you are a parent that you realize how innocent and beautiful every child is... no kid deserves to be bullied. The fact that people are different is what makes the world such a beautiful place. Could you imagine a world where everybody looked or acted the exact same? It would be *horribly* boring! I guess it's true, the older you get, the wiser you become. It's not until I became older that I really realize this, but now that I do recognize how bad bullying is,

I'm going to do my best to make sure my kids don't become bullies. I'm going to try and encourage both to embrace the fact that nobody is the same, and *that's* what makes us all so beautiful. If my son or daughter end up being judged by the outside world and feel like they don't belong, it will crush me. So, no matter what they are dealing with on the outside, I want them knowing they always have a safe place to come home to that's free of judgment. From the second I drove my son home from the hospital, I made it my mission to create a home environment where my kids feel comfortable, safe, and loved. I want them to know I will never judge them, only LOVE them. Another thing that happened while I was driving home from the hospital is I inadvertently was *promoted* to my dream job. There is a saying that "If you do what you love, you'll never have to work a day in your life." I can honestly say that being a father doesn't feel like work. I love every second of it. Sure, there are good days and bad days. There have been days when my kids cry, whine and frustrate the shit out of me, but for as many frustrating days, there have been hundreds more good days. See, for as easy as it is for our kids to piss us off, they can just as easily melt our hearts. My son and daughter figured this out quickly. They both understand that when they give someone a kiss, it was a good thing, so anytime they would do something bad and I would discipline them, they both would immediately run up to me and give me a kiss. It was like a get-out-of-jail-free card. It actually makes disciplining my kids difficult because when they do end up doing something wrong, they look so damn cute doing it.

I think everyone on earth yearns to feel relevant. We want to make our mark on this planet, and that's why I might have been a little reluctant to become a dad. In America, we have a tendency to measure our relevance by our material possessions. It's our outward expression of wealth that shows the people around us that we've made it. We put so much emphasis on our jobs and the size of our bank accounts that we forget about the most important thing: family. In America we have it ass-backwards. We put more emphasis on our careers than we do our relationships. Just look at the divorce statistics if you think I'm wrong.

A few years before I had my son, my wife and I traveled to Guatemala. Since my wife's parents are from Guatemala, my wife had a strong urge to visit there. I was not really keen on going because I'm not all that crazy about third-world countries, but I took one for the team and went with my wife. The first thing I noticed was how poor everybody was and how technology was *non-existent*. We would drive through these small towns called "pueblos" and all you would see were run-down shacks with dirt floors. Now, the first few days, I felt bad for those people living in poverty, but the more time I spent in Guatemala, the more I grew to admire its culture. Where I live, and I think it's probably true for most neighborhoods in America, when people come home from work, we usually walk inside, eat dinner, turn on the TV and relax. There isn't much interaction between neighbors. Outside, most American neighborhoods are ghost towns after seven p.m. because everybody is inside their houses watching TV or looking down at their Smartphone's like zombies. But in third-world countries, it's much different. People don't have the luxury of entertaining themselves with TV or smartphones, so they are forced to interact with one another. When we drove through the different pueblos at night in Guatemala, the streets where alive with people. Nobody was inside, everybody was outside! Open air churches where alive with people singing, kids were kicking balls and playing tag, elders gathered around fires and talked. Even though the Guatemalan people were poor in material things, they were rich in relationships, and I left there admiring them for that. I don't really know why I told the story of Guatemala. I guess it's just to say that as I write this book, and as I continue to raise my children, I hope that I can instill in them the realization that it's the relationships in our lives that make us rich, not the size of our bank accounts.

# WHAT HAPPENED TO
# MY WIFE'S BODY

One of the beautiful things about pregnancy is the woman gets an overnight boob job. I think my wife's breasts grew three-fold; it was awesome. And hard, wow, were they hard! But it's a double-edged sword. Yeah, the woman's boobs are going to be bigger, but it comes at a cost. They are now filled with milk and the breasts become property of baby. My wife was cool and she would let me suck on her breasts but, at first, there was something weird about it. I couldn't get over the fact that I was sucking on the same things that my son was eating from. We'd have sex, but I had to be careful because if I squeezed too hard, I'd get squirted in the face with nature's nectar. Over time, I ended up embracing the breast milk, and it didn't bother me at all. But once the milk stops, bye-bye boobies. It's like one of the Three Stooges pops them with a needle and down they go. So, the once beautiful, hard boobs are now more like half-filled water balloons.

Another body part that I saw get affected was her tummy. During the pregnancy, the woman gets a dark line that runs up from the vagina all the way to the bellybutton. It's not ugly, it's just weird. I don't see a reason for it, and I don't know why it happens, but once the baby is out, the woman's stomach has an interesting rubbery 'Jello-like' texture. Imagine a basketball inside the stomach, stretching the skin for nine months then, all of sudden, the basketball is gone. The woman's belly becomes a jiggly blob. And the skin is wrinkled like an old lady's ass. For the most part, if you give the stomach enough time, it sorta bounces back into shape. But the reality is, unless the women gets a "mommy-tuck", the belly just isn't going to be the same, at least that was the case for us.

My wife's butt never grew like other pregnant girl's butts. I was a little disappointed actually. I fancy myself an "ass-man," so it would have been nice having a little more junk in the trunk. My wife's butt looks the same today as it did before she was pregnant. My friends think I'm a lucky bastard, and when I compare my wife's rearend to some of their wives' butts, I am indeed lucky! But none-the-less, it would have been nice to play with a bigger ass for a few months.

This brings me to the vagina. There are a lot of questions about what happens to the vagina after a vaginal delivery. I'm happy to report that my wife's vagina still feels like a vagina. Many guys think that once a woman gives birth it will feel looser. Here's the strange thing, my wife tore a little bit "down there" when she was pushing out our son, so the doctor stitched her up. I think when the doctor stitched her up, she must have made it tighter. Because when we started having sex again, for several weeks it was like having sex with a virgin. It was tight for me and it hurt her, so we had to be careful the first few months. Once we commenced having sex again, it was a slow, gradual process to stretch her vagina back into form.

These imperfections that happen to the woman's body as a result of giving birth are my wife's badges of honor. It's the ribbon given to her when she became a mother. Personally, I don't mind that my wife's body changed. Actually, I think it's pretty sexy. Those small imperfections are hot to me. I told my wife on several occasions that I thought she was just as beautiful after pregnancy as she was before.

# THE DREADED DIRTY DIAPER

Let me put you as ease, changing a dirty diaper isn't all that bad. Like I mentioned before, the baby's poop doesn't even really smell for the first several months. Through the entire time both my kids were in diapers, I had no problem changing them. It's a lot like when your kid pukes on you. When it's your own kid's fecal matter, it's no big deal. I'll put it to you like this... do you mind the smell of your own poop when you go to the bathroom? For me, the answer is no. Your kid's poop is a bit like yours. You're not going to mind it all that much. Don't get me wrong, there are going to be some pretty fowl diapers that will stink up the entire house, but those are few and far between. I remember gagging a time or two, but I never once thought that changing a dirty diaper was all that bad. It's just part of being a parent. What's the alternative? Not putting diapers on your kid? That would be horrible. I once saw a documentary where a baby in a small village in Africa pooped on the mom, and all the mom did was wipe the poop off her leg with a dried-out piece of corn on the cob. It was amazing how nonchalant the mother was when her kid just pooped on her, and the fact that she didn't care at all is even more amazing. I'm not that big on my kid pooping all over my legs or on my carpet, so I welcome the fact that diapers were invented to make my life easier.

The main thing about changing diapers is that once people have babies, it becomes the mission of the parents to keep baby happy and healthy. All you want to do as a parent is make sure your kid is comfortable, so the second you notice your kid needs a new diaper, you don't even think about the smell. All you care about is getting your son or daughter into a clean diaper, so they don't get a rash. The mission of the parent is to keep the baby's bottom as clean and dry as possible. When a baby's butt is exposed to a soiled diaper for an extended period of time, that's when rashes can happen. I was a big user of baby powder. I thought it did a great job of drying my son and daughter's butts and help fend off rashes. But since that time of me using baby powder, some convincing medical research is out there saying how bad talc powder actually is for us. Apparently, talc can cause cancer! Thanks for the warning label Johnson & Johnson! Since I stopped using talc, Johnson & Johnson has had to pay out serious settlement money to people that developed cancer. As I've become more educated in the world of talc, I would recommend you avoid it. There are some more holistic powders out there that use corn starch that I think might be safer for baby. I guess it all comes down to moderation. Using baby powder with talc every now and then shouldn't hurt your kid. I used it for a majority of both my kids' time in diapers and they seem to be just fine. But if you can avoid talc, I would.

# I HAVE TO WAIT HOW LONG TO HAVE SEX AGAIN?

So, after the woman gives birth, sex is going to be off limits for a while. I think I had to wait over eight weeks before my wife and I were able to make love again. Now before you (guys) start freaking out, I can guarantee, that at some point in your life, you went through a dry spell for longer than eight weeks. Hell, I bet most of you guys have gone six or more *months* without getting any action while you were single, so waiting eight weeks for the woman who just bore your child is really no big deal. In the meantime, there are plenty of ways a couple can have fun together in the bedroom other than having intercourse. Wait, who am I kidding? There won't be any time for sex the first eight weeks, so don't worry about that little waiting period. My wife and I were so busy getting acclimated to being new parents and the learning curve that goes with it that the thought of sex was the furthest thing from our minds. The first eight weeks are pretty exhausting... fun... but exhausting. It's really all about rhythm. After a few days, my wife and I got in a rhythm of taking care of both of our kids. Our kids naturally found their sleep patterns and eating times. We didn't force it on them, we just found that it developed organically.

# WHAT DO I FEED THIS KID?

There are many choices and formulas out there that you can give your kid. I was pretty stressed about the food thing. I wanted to make sure my kid was getting the best nutrition humanly possible. Fortunately, my wife was one of the lucky moms to have their breastmilk come in. What I come to find out, breast milk isn't a given. Some moms don't produce it. My wife and I went to nursing classes, and there were moms in there that had bottles of formula attached to these bra contraptions pretending like they were breastfeeding. I didn't know what to think of that really. I thought it was a little weird, but who am I to tell a mom what to do with her kid. If she wants to experience the gift of breastfeeding, then more power to her. If your partner does produce breastmilk, my advice would be to give it to your kid. Why? Because it will save you a shit load of money for starters. Why go buy something when nature gives it to you for free? It's like buying bottled water when the free stuff comes out of the faucet. Okay, scratch that, it's like buying sand if you live at the beach. Doesn't make sense. Not only that, but it's nature's perfect nectar. Babies have been living and growing off of breastmilk since the beginning of man, so why change that? Nature knows what it's doing, and if it produces a food naturally for babies chances are it's some pretty good shit. Our doctor told us that breastmilk didn't have any Vitamin D in it, so we were supposed to give our kids drops of Vitamin D as a supplement. To be honest, I bought the Vitamin D, but my wife and I were pretty bad about giving it to our kids every day. It's not like we didn't want to, we would just forget. I actually think I ended up spilling a bottle or two along the way also. I think for me, I wasn't as strict about giving my kids the Vitamin D because my thought is that if nature wanted it in there, nature would have put it in there. I don't know what Vitamin D is good for, so it's really up to you and your doctor if you want to go through the added expense of buying a supplement for your kid at such a young age. My kids didn't get the Vitamin D on a regular basis, and they turned out just fine, so for me, the verdict is still out as to whether or not Vitamin D is really that much of a necessity. Again, I think if nature wanted the babies to have it, nature probably would have put it in the breastmilk. If your partner can't produce breastmilk or doesn't want to deal with it, don't worry about it. Your kid is going to grow up just fine on the store-bought variety. My wife stopped producing breastmilk at about nine months for my son and at about six months for my daughter, so we had to transition them both onto formula. They both transitioned without a hitch, but I will tell you that my son only would drink the premixed liquid variety, while my daughter was fine with the powder. It's crazy how picky babies can be at such a young age, but I guess at even only a few weeks old, they know what they like. I believe the powder variety is a bit cheaper, so if you can get your kid to like the powder stuff, you're probably going to save some money along the way. Whether it's powder formula or liquid, know that both smell like a sweaty sock you've left in your gym bag for two weeks. I don't know how babies drink it, and I don't know why formula companies don't figure out a way to make it taste and smell better. I guess they don't have to make it smell good because the baby doesn't know any better. I'm a big proponent of organic. I don't know if it's really organic, or if it's just a label they put on there to make us *think* it's organic, but I ended up choosing an organic formula for both my kids. I think it's important to try to feed your kid as natural of an ingredient as possible, considering so much of that energy is used to grow.

# WILL YOU PLEASE
# SHUT UP!?

When I think back to before I was a dad, I would cringe at the sound of a baby crying. I couldn't imagine why nature would produce such an annoying sound. Even at church, when I should be forgiving and thinking about God, if a heard a baby cry, I would curse that crying baby out in my head. On airplane flights, it would take *real* restraint to keep me from telling a parent to shut their crying kid up. It sounds weird, but when you become a parent, your response to the sound of a baby's cry changes. It becomes less annoying. And, as a matter of fact, you actually become more sympathetic to a baby's cry. There's not a baby in the world that doesn't cry, so there's not a parent in the world that hasn't had to deal with a crying baby. Every parent in the world knows that the first thing you do as a parent is to try and stop a baby from crying and, sometimes, no matter what you do, the baby simply *won't stop crying.* I am way more sympathetic to parents flying with kids now. I know that you are under a hundred times more stress traveling with kids than traveling without kids. The second I hear a crying baby on an airplane, I actually smile because I know that most people on that plane were once in that position themselves. There was one instance where my wife and I were traveling with my son, and we didn't prepare him a bottle for takeoff. We thought, based on his normal eating schedule, we would have time to make a bottle for him once we got in the air. Well, we ended up getting caught on the tarmac, *and* got held up on the ground for longer than expected. My son got cranky, and he would not stop crying. My wife and I were horrified because in that moment, I was with "the crying baby on an airplane." My wife rocked my son, she shushed him, I gave him every single toy that we had in our carry-on, and *nothing* was stopping him from crying. I felt terrible, but then an elderly lady sitting across the aisle started shaking a box of *Tic Tacs* in front of my son's face. For a brief moment, he stopped crying. It was something he'd never seen or heard before. The lady smiled and handed me the box of *Tic Tacs*. As the woman handed me the *Tic Tacs*, I could see compassion in her face. I knew that she knew exactly what we were going through. It comforted me knowing I wasn't the only person in the world that has had to deal with a crying baby on an airplane. Every time I travel, I'll never forget that moment, and it reminds me to have sympathy for others traveling with small kids.

The important thing to remember about crying is all the baby is really doing is calling you -- and nine times out of ten, once you pick baby up or give them what they need, they will stop crying. Both my kids had different cries. They had an "I'm hungry" cry, they had an "I'm tired" cry, and they had a "I've got a dirty diaper" cry. No two babies' cries are the same, I can tell you that! Within an hour of my son's birth, I could differentiate his cry from other babies in the hospital. I remember a specific instance when I was walking back to our postpartum room. I had left the room to get my wife some juice (a little off track, but the hospital we stayed in had the best juice I'd ever tasted), and the nurse told me they had a juice machine, and they would mix a few of the juices together. I think it was orange, apple, and tropical fruit mixed together. Anyway, as I walked back from getting my wife this ridiculously good juice, I heard several babies crying down the hallway from various postpartum rooms. I specifically made a mental note, and was surprised to realize that they all sounded different. It was like a veil had been lifted off of my ears, and I now had this "sixth-sense" of being able to differentiate baby voices. There were probably six babies crying in various postpartum rooms, and I knew with 100% certainty that none of those crying babies was my son. I was shocked to discover that babies *actually* sound different from one another. Even though baby is not saying any words, he or she is still talking to you. I liken a baby's cry to fingerprints; I believe no two are alike. Each baby has a unique sound that is exclusive to them. It doesn't take long for parents to hone in on their kid's unique sound. Before I was a parent, I'd tell you that all crying babies sounded alike, but now I *completely* disagree with that. If ten babies were crying, I can, without seeing them, 100%, tell you if one of those crying babies is my son or daughter. I could hear both my kids cry from across the room. Not because they were loud, but because I *recognized* their voices. It makes sense really. It's no different than when somebody you know calls you on the telephone. My wife doesn't have to tell me her name every time she calls me for me to know it's her. Babies are no different. Even at a couple hours old, babies already have their own unique voice. Even though babies are not speaking with words, the fact is that they are still speaking. And it's easy for a parent to recognize his or her baby's cry. You'll get to know your kid's cry *really* quickly, and you'll see… it's not that annoying.

A baby cries for one purpose, they want "something." Babies don't cry to piss us parents off (although sometimes it might feel that way), a baby cries to simply say, "Hey, Mom… Dad, a little help over here!" Within the first few weeks of meeting baby, parents quickly get a grasp for what their little one wants.

Now, a baby crying doesn't *nearly* annoy me as much as a whining baby. Babies cry only when they are really unhappy. But if they are bored or just generally not having a good time, they whine. Whining pisses me off because they are just being brats. Crying I get. They are hungry, wet diaper, sick. But when they whine, they are just being punks or divas. My son whined a lot in the house. He wasn't hot, he wasn't cold, he wasn't hungry, and he wasn't tired. He was bored. My son would whine until I took him outside. As soon as he was outside, cool as a cucumber. Whining was my son's way of saying, "I'm sick of playing with the toys, Dad… house is too small… take me somewhere… challenge me intellectually." As much as it annoyed me when my son whined, looking back, it was really kinda cool. It's fascinating to me that at such a young age, his little brain demanded more. He wanted to see what was outside. See, a baby's brain is like a sponge, and they constantly need to be stimulated. Before I became a parent, I used to think babies were just blobs that didn't think or speak. However, as I was able to watch my son and daughter grow up, I witnessed just how smart a baby *actually* is. They might not have the ability to communicate with words, but I promise, *they will communicate*. And everything they say to you is direct, and it is specific to *exactly* what they want or need. Just by the simple act of walking outside, my son's brain was bombarded with all this "eye candy." Instead of staring at the wall, he was looking at cars, trees, and birds. His brain couldn't get enough of it. I think that's why so many kids enjoy going for walks in strollers. Both my son and daughter *loved* to go on walks. I think, for starters, that it gets *everybody* out of the house. But really, I'm absolutely convinced that my kids loved walks because their little brains were able to take in their surroundings and give the brain the stimuli it needed for them to learn.

# I'M A WALKING ZOMBIE

You'll hear this a lot during the pregnancy: "Get a lot of sleep, you'll need it". First of all, sleep isn't something you can store up like a spare battery you can call upon at a moment's notice. Sleep is individual to each day, so the fact that people tell you to get your rest is just plain stupid. I will tell you to enjoy those last few days of sleeping in because those days will be *long gone* once baby arrives. Both my kids are good sleepers, but sleeping in just isn't in their vocabulary. I keep telling them sleep is okay, but both my son and daughter wake up early. I'm convinced they think they are going to miss something. As much as it's frustrating to get woken up every morning, it starts to become intoxicating. I can't tell you how awesome it is to be woken up by my beautiful daughter gabbing my finger and saying, "Daddy, get up!" or my four-year-old son coming in the room yelling, "Daddy, look! I'm wearing boxers, just like you!" Having the blessing of starting your day by being greeted with pure love and innocence is beyond words, and I can tell you *that* I'm going to miss it. I know that soon my kids won't storm into my room the second they get up. Soon, my kids will be grown up, and I won't be the center of their attention, but as long as they are young, and I'm that person they hold high on a pedestal, I'm going to try and embrace every early morning with zest and excitement because my kids' first instinct in the morning is to wake me up. Every morning, as much as I want to go back to bed, I can't say "No" to either of their beautiful little faces. I've learned a lot from my kids, probably more than they've learned from me, so I don't blame them for not wanting to sleep, they simply don't want to miss the joys of life.

But in those first several months, I can absolutely say, sleep will be at a premium. It's true that you kinda live your life in a fog. One day, I actually left the house to go to the gym, and I was wearing just boxers. I got in my car and looked down and realized I had forgotten to put on my shorts. The first few months without sleep are just that, a few months. You get through it just like every parent before you has, so don't expect a medal because you went to work on just one hour's sleep. It's your job to take care of your kid and relish in every late night you get with them. I promise you, you will look back on those nights, and one day wish your kid was a baby again, sleeping on your shoulder in the middle of the night.

# SCHEDULE? WHAT SCHEDULE?

I read a lot of books and got a lot of advice from parents who've told me about the importance of putting my kid on a strict eating and sleeping schedule. I challenge any parent-to-be to write down a schedule they would *like* to keep... and try to keep it. Taking care of a baby is a lot like life. You roll with the punches. My wife and I had fantasies about what our dream schedule would be, but the fact of the matter is that the *baby* dictates the schedule. One day he or she might wake up at five, another day at four. Most of the time it's predictable, but sometimes it isn't, so don't go freaking out if baby waits an hour to eat; maybe the little guy or girl isn't hungry. If baby skips a meal, chances are they'll make it up later in the day. Baby will fall into its own rhythm of how it likes to do things, and you just have to go with what makes baby happy. Don't stress about finding that schedule or rhythm right out of the gate. It will take a few weeks of getting to know your baby before you get a handle on how they like things.

# QUIET TIME BEFORE BED

Once parenthood begins, there will be a few hours each day that you'll tend to cherish, at least I do. It's the few hours between putting the kids to bed and when you and your partner go to bed. Those hours of the day have come to be my most relaxing. It's not because there is finally some peace and quiet around the house. For me, it is more the fact that I know my son and daughter are safe and peacefully sleeping in their beds. I know nothing is going to happen to them. I know they aren't getting into trouble or climbing on something that can hurt them. I just know they are safe. And knowing your kids are safe is one of the most relaxing feelings that can take over your body. I tend to be a little overly paranoid. Whether I like it or not, I'm always analyzing a location or situation and thinking of worst case scenarios. When my kids are at the park, I'm always thinking and visualizing all the ways they can get hurt, so I'd say that a majority of the day, when my kids are awake, I'm *completely* stressed out -- always following them around, making sure they don't hurt themselves. I have this obsessive brain that's always trying to think of worst case scenarios before they happen, in hopes that nothing bad will ever happen to my kids. I know it's completely bullshit, and I can never anticipate *all* the bad stuff that can happen, but I can't help being obsessed about my kid's safety. So, I think that's why those few hours between when my kids go to bed and when my wife and I go to bed, I'm the most relaxed. I know they are in their beds, and I know they are safe. I actually have a similar relaxation when I get in the car. In the early going, both my son and daughter didn't particularly care for their car seats, so the first few months they were born, it was stressful at times taking them in the car because they would cry and there wasn't anything we could really do about it. But over time, both my kids became acclimated to the car, and they stopped all the crying. Once my kids liked being in the car, the car became a very relaxing place for me. It all goes back to the safety thing. I know when I place my kids in their car seats, they can't go anywhere. They are strapped in and in a safe place. I know anything can happen in a car and accidents can happen, but for some reason, when my kids are in their car seats, I'm relaxed. I also have some of the greatest little conversations with my kids in the car. It's a moment in time when we are all trapped in the same small space. We are usually okay with being trapped in that space, so we all just take the opportunity to relax and talk to each other. My daughter, who is two now as I write this, has a thing about always taking off her shoes. She laughs and rips her shoes and socks off as soon as she's in the car. It used to get on our nerves, but over time it became a joke. We knew as soon as she sat down and we started driving, we'd hear laughing, saying, "Shoes off, Daddy!", and then we playfully joke with her that her shoes are off. God, as I sit and write this, I'm already starting to miss when these days will come to an end. It's these little moments between moments that makes being a parent so great.

Those few hours between baby being put down to sleep and your own bedtime is also a really good time for Mom and Dad to reconnect. The busyness of the day is gone, whether that be work or baby, and it's time to unwind. This is when my wife and I usually pop a bottle of wine, talk, and watch TV. Now that I think about it, it seems to be a pretty relaxing time for my dog too. For the 12 hours prior, he was being relentlessly harassed by my two kids, so he seems really relaxed during these few hours too. My dog would usually jump on my lap and go into a very relaxing, deep sleep. For a few hours each day, when the kids are in bed, it's almost like you revert back to not having any kids. The house is quiet. You're relaxed. It's just a reprieve from the hustle and bustle. Now, if eight weeks have passed and Mom's vagina is back in business, this is also a great time to fit in some hanky-panky. With kids comfortably asleep, the entire house is fair game. You can have sex on the couch, on the floor, or in the kitchen. Just be careful what you're doing because it only takes one bottle of wine, a frisky night of watching TV, and you'll be out looking for bunk beds.

# Get Away from Me, Dog

I'm a dog lover, always have been. I grew up with German Shepherds and they were everything to me. My favorite dog growing up was named Leo. Leo was huge black German Shepherd with two small patches of tan on his cheeks. When I walked down the street with him, people would cross to the other side because Leo was so intimidating. Cool thing was, Leo looked like he would tear your head off, but he wouldn't hurt a fly. He was a big teddy bear, so when my wife and I got together and she wanted a dog, I told my wife German Shepherds were the only dogs I would ever own. Two weeks later, we brought home a pug. Yeah, I didn't win that battle. The wife wanted a pug, and she got one. No masculine German Shepherd for this guy, instead I got a small fat dog with a squished face. When I first found out my wife wanted a pug, the first thing that went through my head was, "What an ugly dog. Why on earth would anybody want such a hideous looking animal?" It's like God whacked all the pugs of the world in the face with a frying pan, and sent them on their way. There's absolutely no reason for a dog to have a squished snout. It brings on a whole litany of medical problems. For starters, pugs can't breathe well, they overheat quickly, they snore, and they constantly have issues with their eyes, skin and ears. If you give pugs wet food, they have to bury their heads in the bowl to get every bite and end up wearing half the food in the bowl. Pugs are so fat and their snouts are so short, they try like bloody hell to reach their balls, but it's no use. They always fall a good six inches short. I feel sorry for my pug; his balls are like dangling a carrot in front of him. You see it in his eyes, he wants so badly to lick his junk, but he just can't reach.

Well, when we first brought our pug home, I didn't think I would ever like him. I was too big and masculine to have a wimpy, fat dog. He just didn't fit into what I felt a dog represented. It wasn't even an hour after picking him up that I fell head over heels in love with him. As big and macho as I claim to be, I still have a soft heart. And the second I held that dog, my heart melted. I was putty in his paws. I took him everywhere with me. Originally, the idea behind the dog was that he would be my wife's, but that plan got thrown out the window once I took a liking to him. Overnight, I became obsessed with our pug, and he became my new best friend. I was so whacked out in love with this dog that I turned into one of those people that I once loathed. I actually let my dog sit on my lap when I was driving. I used to hate those people, and now... I had become one. When I flew to Chicago to visit family, my pug was laying under the seat in front of me on the plane. I bought my dog birthday and Christmas presents. I loved him with everything I had and he loved me. My wife and I found ourselves having friends with pugs, and we would have puppy play dates. We would get the dogs together, so they could play. How ridiculous is that!? For several years, I can honestly say, our dog was our kid.

Well, my brother had two kids before me, and when I would visit him in Chicago, he would always laugh at me and tell me that once I had a real kid of my own, my feelings for my dog would change. I didn't believe him. In that moment, I didn't think there was *anything* in the world that could change my feelings toward my dog. I didn't understand how the love for a child could negate the love I already had for my dog. Well, when my son came along, and just like my brother said, my dog went from chief of the tribe to low man on the totem pole. It's not that I didn't love my dog anymore because I did and still do. However, my view of him shifted. He's still a part of the family, but his role has changed. He's no longer a kid, but rather just "the dog."

To get our dog acclimated to having a baby in the house, we were given some tips from friends on what to do before you bring baby in the house. I don't know if they work, but it's what we did and it made sense to us. Everybody knows dogs rely heavily on their sense of smell, so before we brought my son into the house, I went into the house alone and brought him an article of clothing baby was wearing. I let my pug smell the article of clothing before my son was brought into the house. The article of clothing we decided to go with was the bonnet they put on my son the second he was born. I felt like that had the most opportunity for scents for my dog to pick up on. It's a little gross, but the bonnet actually had remanence of crusty baby juices left over from when my son was born. I figured the more scents the better. So, the day we got home from the hospital, my wife and son stayed in the car while I went into the house to introduce our dog to our son's scents. My dog was certainly curious of the hat and sniffed it. Once I felt my dog had gotten from the hat what he needed, I put the dog on the leash and walked him outside and introduced him to my son. I thought it better that my dog and son meet outside the house, that way the dog wouldn't think my son was invading his turf. I let my dog sniff my son outside and, once the introduction was complete, we all walked into the house together like one big family. It might sound a little cheesy, but I thought it was important and symbolic to the dog that we were not replacing him, but simply adding to our family dynamic. And as corny as it sounds, I wanted my dog to feel like he was welcoming our son into the house at the same time we were. Having the introduction happen outside of the home was important to me. Whether it worked or not, I don't know, but I do believe my dog accepted my son with open paws. I've never had an issue with jealously *or* aggression. And my son and dog became good friends. When my daughter was born, I did the same thing. It's amazing how dogs pick up on the little things. Before my son was born, my dog would get excited when I grabbed his leash because he knew he was going for a walk. Now, my dog jumps up with excitement when I put a jacket on my son or daughter. My dog was smart enough to observe that when I put a jacket on my son or daughter that meant I'm going to walk them around the neighborhood in the stroller. In the end, my dog's life might have gotten better in some respect because we do take him for longer walks sometimes. It isn't just the "hurry and take a shit walk." Sometimes I'll take my son for a good hour-and-a-half walk, so the dog has benefited a little from my kids being around. The other amazing thing about dogs, at least with mine, is he keeps to himself during the day. It's almost like my dog knows that my son and daughter come first, so he doesn't even bother us. All of our attention has to be geared toward the kids, so the dog has adjusted his lifestyle to accommodate that. But what's cool is when my son and daughter go down to sleep at night, my dog almost instantly jumps off of the other couch and jumps on either my lap or my wife's. It's like he knows that my kids are now sleeping, and it's my dog's time to get some much needed love. Being a dog owner, I wouldn't change it. Sure, there is more bullshit you have to deal with, and they can cost you a bunch of cash sometimes, but I like having the companionship of a dog, and I think the advantages *far* outweigh the negatives. I grew up a dog owner and I want my kids to have that same experience.

A little side-note on dogs. They welcome the snack of a warm shitty diaper. One time I was trying to multitask, and I had just changed my kid's poopy diaper and I threw it in the garbage. I took the garbage bag out of the trashcan with the intention of throwing the bag full of soiled diapers away outside. For whatever reason, dealing with the kid and doing other stuff, I forgot that I'd placed the full bag of diapers on the floor of my son's room. I left the house to drop my son off at Grandma's for the day. Well, my wife got home before I did, and when she opened the front door she was greeted with the house smelling like shit. My dog had ripped into the garbage bag and ate a couple poopy diapers. I didn't see it, but apparently it was disgusting. My dog had decided to dine on the shitty diapers comfortably nuzzled on our sofa. Baby poop was smeared all over the couch. My wife was scrubbing the couch for several hours that day. Her exact quote to me was, "I wasn't planning on doing this today." Before you think it's just my nasty dog that eats baby diapers… they all do it. I've got two friends and a brother that can back up my story with stories of their own.

# IS MY KID BREATHING?

One of the joys of parenting that many people don't talk about is the paranoia surrounding your kid's breathing. As soon as your baby is born, you're going to constantly be checking if he or she is still breathing. I don't know why we parents constantly check to see if our baby is breathing, but we just do. The first night in the hospital, I remember not sleeping a wink. I was constantly getting up from my cot to make sure my son's tiny lungs were doing what they were supposed to be doing. I don't really think there was any real reason to have this paranoia. Nobody in the hospital seemed to be worried that my son would all of a sudden stop breathing, but I couldn't help it. I was obsessed with making sure he was breathing. I guess it's just part of becoming a new parent. There's a condition called SIDS, when babies suddenly die in their sleep for no apparent reason. I think that helped put the fear of God in me, so I was constantly worried about my son and daughter. There were actually a few times when my son was in such a deep sleep that I poked him. He wasn't too happy being woken up, but I was happy he was still breathing. For the first time in my life, I was responsible for a life, and I think it was normal for me to always make sure my kids were okay. Breathing is the first indicator that life is present, so checking to see if baby is breathing is a natural response to being a new parent. Even to this day, I make sure both my kids are breathing. If we are in the car and one of them is sleeping in their child seat, I'll make sure I see them breathing. Or, if they're asleep in the stroller, I'll bend down and focus my attention on their chest. If I see their chests moving, all is okay in the world.

# CHILDPROOFING THE DIGS

When I found out we were having a baby, I thought I had to have the house childproofed as soon as we brought baby home from the hospital. Come to find out, that's not the case. Childproofing doesn't come into play until the kid is at least six months old. It doesn't matter before that because the kid can't move anywhere. He's a prisoner in his or her own body. Where you lay baby down is where they stay. But once your kid starts moving, I promise it will be like a tornado went off in the house, and you'll miss the days of dropping them in a swing so you can get a load of laundry done.

As far as the actual childproofing, look for the obvious things that can hurt your kid. Babies are going to want to grab *everything*. When I say everything, I mean *everything*. Nothing goes unnoticed by a baby. If there is something that isn't a toy, and it's within arms-reach, they'll grab it. And kids are great at finding stuff. If you lose your car keys and have been looking all over for them, set your kid loose around the house, and I bet he or she finds them in five minutes. Babies have a knack for finding shit we adults don't even know is there. It's actually quite awesome to watch. Watching the baby's brain develop and observing their curiosity was one of my favorite parts of watching my son and daughter grow up. Babies are so eager to learn, and it fascinated me to watch my kids' little brains soak up their surroundings like a sponge.

Anchoring down light furniture is a *must* when child proofing a home. The second babies start standing up, they immediately crawl to a piece of furniture for leverage. If you have a lightweight end-table or bookcase, bolt that thing to the wall, so it doesn't fall on baby. Corners are another big worry. If you go to a baby store, they have foam corners that you can tape on the edges of tables. Just know that the tape that comes in the package sucks, and your little one will spot the foam corner and rip that bad boy right off the end-table. My foam corners lasted about 12 hours before my son ripped them off and was chewing on them. I didn't even put them on the corners for my daughter because I knew they wouldn't last. Keep a look out for glass. My entertainment center had two doors on the front that had glass inserts. It made me nervous that my son might fall and smash his head into the glass pane, so I went to the local hardware store and replaced the glass with Plexiglass. That reverts back to my obsession with visualizing the worst-case scenario in every room. I doubt most parents would think to replace their glass doors on their entertainment system with Plexiglass, but it was a necessity for me. My entertainment center kept the same look, but I had the peace of mind, knowing that if my son smashed his head into the Plexiglass, it wasn't going to shatter and cut him.

Babyproofing the kitchen is a big one. Usually there are tons of chemicals under the sink that you don't want baby getting into, so securing that cabinet door is a *must*. The other main reason to make sure the cabinet doors don't open is baby is going to use the door for leverage to stand up. They use their little hands to grab onto the handle to pull themselves up. If the door isn't secured and closed, it will swing open on baby and they could get hurt. I learned a trick: give your kid a cabinet because they like digging through stuff, and it will keep them occupied while you cook. Basically, you allocate one cabinet they can dig through, and fill it with plastic *Tupperware*. They can't hurt themselves with the *Tupperware*, and letting them dig through a cabinet might keep them occupied enough so you can cook dinner.

I didn't do much to childproof the bathroom. I just moved the chemicals to a place my kids couldn't reach them. I've heard of parents childproofing the toilet; I don't think that's a bad idea, I just didn't do it. I didn't want my kid in the bathroom, period, so I kept the bathroom door closed so they couldn't get in there. I thought it was gross for them to be crawling around on the bathroom floor. To me, there was something nasty about that. As my wife can attest, I don't exactly have the best aim when it comes to hitting the toilet. I have been known to get a couple drops here and there on the floor, so I *really* didn't want my kid crawling through that stuff. For me, the best way to keep my crawling kids out of the bathroom was to close the door.

## ON THE MOVE

I think what makes the house messy once baby starts crawling is the fact that you can never leave them alone from that point on. It's not like babies throw their toys all over the place, it's more the fact that you don't have time to pick anything up. And by anything, I mean anything. I feel like once my kids started crawling, there was tons of shit all over the house. My wife's shoes, my shoes, jackets, sweatshirts, dishes, you name it, it was spread all over the house. The house is messy because you constantly have to follow baby around, and you don't have much free time to get stuff done around the house. If you turn your head for *literally* a second, baby can get into something that could possibly harm them. One day, I left my kid in the living-room for no more than ten seconds. I think I went into the kitchen to grab a glass of water. When I returned, I saw him playing with something in his mouth. I put my finger in his mouth and pulled out a penny. No harm, no foul. But, it scared the shit out of me. I started thinking "what if". What if he swallowed the penny, and God forbid he started choking. I wouldn't have been able to live with myself. So once the little one does become mobile, make sure you always have eyes on them and constantly scan the floors for loose change that might have fallen out of your pocket. It goes back to the fact that if it's on the floor, a baby will find it. I inadvertently dropped a penny from my pants, and it could have gone bad, but thankfully it didn't.

## Hospital Tests

There are a bunch of tests the hospital performs on kids once they are born. Most all the tests involve drawing blood. They are testing for various disorders and for jaundice.

Jaundice is when there is excess bilirubin in the baby's bloodstream. I don't know why some babies have excess bilirubin, but if they do, they usually look yellow. The way the doctors fix this is by throwing some sunglasses on your kid, and laying them under an ultraviolet light. Both my kids checked out okay, so they didn't have to go through it. But I know a lot of parents whose child *did* have jaundice. From what I gather, it's pretty common, and it's nothing to freak out about. I don't know if every state has the same tests, but I feel California has a bunch. One test, in particular, really needed a lot of blood, as far as I was concerned. They pricked my kids on the heel and squeezed the shit out of their foot for what felt like ten minutes, all so they could put enough blood on a sheet of paper for the test to be performed. For some blood tests, you'll get the results right away, like if his or her iron is low, but some of the other tests go off to a lab, so the state can perform the test and you only get notified if something is wrong. So, no news is good news as far as the tests are concerned. The other test they are going to perform is a hearing test. I don't know how the hell they check a baby's hearing if the baby can't tell you whether or not they hear something. But, nonetheless, nurses put sensors on your baby's head and put earphones over their ears. I guess they shoot some sounds through the earphones and the machine picks up on brain activity. If your kid can hear, the brain is going to respond to the sound, and it will show up on the computer. It's some pretty high-tech stuff. Fortunately, both my kids passed all the tests with flying colors. The idea of the tests can be a bit alarming. Not because they are really hurting your baby, but because it "mind fucks" you. You start worrying that your baby might have something wrong with him or her. Chances are, your kid is perfectly fine, so don't let the tests get to you.

# Circumcision

If you're having a boy, you're going to be confronted with a pretty important dilemma. Should I circumcise, or shouldn't I? I think the verdict is still out if you really need to do it. I personally decided to do it because I'm circumcised, and I think an uncircumcised penis looks weird. The procedure itself isn't all that bad. The entire time in the hospital, I didn't leave either of my kid's side. If they had to leave the room for a test, I went with them. The circumcision was no exception. A lot of parents don't want to see their son's penis cut with a knife, so they don't witness it. As for me, I wouldn't dare let my son go through it alone. I wheeled him into the back room where our doctor had a gurney laid out on a counter. When I say gurney, I mean it. It looked like a mini-torture device. It's a plastic mold the size of a baby with Velcro straps that keep the baby from moving around during the procedure. The doctor took my son, strapped him in, and snipped it. The entire procedure didn't take but a few minutes. The doctor uses several tools to make sure they do a good job. I was proud of my son, he took it like a man. He cried a bit, as I expected him to do, but the beautiful thing is… I was there to immediately hold him after it happened. I let him know everything was going to be okay, and he quickly calmed in my arms. The sad thing is, I saw several other babies in there getting circumcised, and they didn't have their dads with them. They had to go at it alone. If you decide to get your son circumcised, I suggest that somebody go in there with him. It's the first few hours of life, and he'll know from the very beginning you'll always be there for him. I later found out that the Vitamin K is essential for this procedure, in order for the blood to clot after the snipping.

Once your son has been snipped, you'll have to take some extra precautions taking care of the penis to ensure it heals properly. The penis is going to be raw for several days, so along with changing the diaper regularly, you have to put a gauze pad with a glob of *Vaseline* over the penis. This helps the area heal and protects the raw tissue from being exposed to the urine. It sounds worse than it is. I did feel like I could tell my son was uncomfortable for a few days, but I don't think it affected his sleep or eating patterns.

Along with the gauze with *Vaseline*, you have to always make sure you pull the remaining skin up and down every time you change the diaper. It's very important you do this because if you don't massage the skin up

and down, the raw tissue will heal by adhering itself
to the head of the penis. If it heals like that, he can't
get an erection without pain or discomfort because the
skin will be too tight. And, yes, babies get erections. My
kid sported "morning wood" on a daily basis. On our
son's three-month check-up, our pediatrician saw that
my son's circumcision did not heal properly, and he
yanked down on the skin, literally tearing it off of the
head of the penis. It was like my son got circumcised all
over again. He was raw and we had to put the *Vaseline*
with gauze on him again. I felt horrible and had some
feelings of guilt for not doing my job as a parent, and
for letting that happen to my son. After all, it was my
responsibility, not his, to make sure his penis healed
properly... and I failed. Our pediatrician made me
feel a little better when he told me he performed that
procedure on eight other babies that day before us.
Our doctor says it's extremely common for the skin
to heal that way. Even though it's common, it doesn't
make it right. Really massage the skin up and down,
so it doesn't attach itself to the head of the penis. You
never want to subject baby to any unnecessary pain
that can easily be avoided.

# TAKE AS MUCH STUFF AS YOU CAN FIT IN YOUR BAG

Hospitals are generous, and they are more than willing to give you the basic necessities to get you rolling in your first few weeks of being parents. Don't be afraid to ask for stuff. I took probably a dozen packages of diapers, and I don't know how many swaddle blankets. I'm not sure if we even had to buy newborn diapers because I snagged so many from the hospital. If you're cool with the nurses, they'll be cool with you and hook you up when the time is right. Now, I don't know if I ended up being charged for those diapers or not because when I got the final hospital bill, it didn't itemize everything and my insurance picked up most the tab. For all I know, I might have paid a hundred dollars per package of diapers.

In addition to diapers, I would recommend grabbing as many of those suction ball contraptions that are used to suck snot out of your kid's nose. The ones they sell at the local pharmacy don't work nearly as well as the ones they have in the hospital. I learned that trick from one of my buddy's wives. There's something about that blue ball that sucks snot like no other. In keeping with the theme of snot, our pediatrician told us about this snot sucking device you can get online. Basically, it's something you stick in your kid's nose that is attached to a tube with a mouthpiece and you literally "suck" the snot out of your kid's nose. I witnessed my wife use it a lot when my kid's nose was stuffy. She would squirt a little bit of saline solution up my kid's nose to loosen up the snot, and then she would suck it out with her mouth. At the end of the day, my wife preferred the devise where she sucked out the snot with her mouth.

If you have a boy and you decide to get him circumcised, be sure to stock up on gauze and *Vaseline*. Hospitals have the perfect size square gauze pieces that work great for applying the *Vaseline* and fitting them under the diaper. I ran out of the gauze squares, and it was hard to find equivalents. Not only that, but I don't know when the last time was that you bought gauze, but it's not cheap. The gauze at the pharmacies is expensive, considering the amount you're getting. And none of the sizes they offer are right for baby.

# DADDY BONDING

As I eluded to before, I don't think that guys bond with the baby the same way the woman does during the pregnancy process. I didn't have this rush of love for him the second I laid eyes on him. It's hard to explain, I knew I loved my son, but I didn't have the obsessed feelings yet that I couldn't live without him. After all, I had lived without him for the 30+ years up until that point, so it's logical that I wasn't madly in love the second I met him, or that I couldn't imagine my life without him. It's very different for your second child because at that point you know what being a parent is all about. You have experienced the love and know what to expect, so when I met my daughter for the first time -- it was *definitely* a different experience than meeting my son. I think I had a much quicker, almost instant connection with my daughter. I think it was purely because I was already a parent in that moment. I'll explain the best I can: the first few months with my son, for me, was the journey of becoming a parent for the first time.

For me, my bond and love with my son grew exponentially, over time, and it really started after he was a few months old. One month after my son was born, I was offered a job out of town that would last several months. So, there I was, a new father, and at only four weeks of my son being on this planet, I was going to have to leave him. I packed up for Boston and left my wife to fend for herself, while I brought home some money. I think this physical distance I had placed between me and my son affected my ability to bond with him. I wasn't with him on a regular basis for months two and three. I flew home, on average, once every two weeks, and the trips were very short-lived. I got home late Friday night, spent all day with my wife and kid Saturday, then flew out sometime Sunday evening. It's hard to bond with somebody when you hardly see him. I can say that as I look back, if I had to leave my son, I'm glad it was in the first couple months of his life. The reality is, whether the dad is around or not, I still think it's hard for Dad to bond with baby in the first few months. The baby really doesn't give any emotional feedback to the dad, acknowledging that the dad exists. In babies' first couple months of life, they are really just blobs. They don't interact with you in the least bit. They don't smile. They don't laugh. They don't even follow you around the room with their eyes. For the first few weeks, babies just stare off into space. For me, during this time, it was still hard for me to bond with my son. I'd talk to him and give him kisses, but there was no reciprocation. I loved him, but he was yet to love me back.

Now, my wife will tell you that her favorite part of being a parent was those first few months. It makes sense, especially for my wife, who breastfed. My son literally needed her to live, so I do feel he was loving her back. He would look at her and almost thank her. There was definitely some sort of connection that was beyond my connection with him. In one particular instance, I remember watching my son feed off my wife. When he was finished, he had this smirk on his face. It was almost like he was saying, "Mom, I don't know what you got in them tits, but man, it's the shit!" He was milk-drunk. You could see it in his eyes, he was wasted and loving every second of it. I've heard stories of dads getting jealous in the early going because they can't give baby what Mom can. I personally didn't feel any jealously. I found the process of watching my son and wife bond quite beautiful. I could see this intense bond forming, and I loved it. I mean, that's what you want. You want your kid to love his or her mom, and you want the mom to love their kids back, so I thought it was great. But I was still waiting for my time. I was still waiting for that feeling parents say they get when they have kids. I was waiting for that warm fuzzy feeling.

As the weeks progressed and they started turning into months, my son started becoming less of a blob. He started following me around the room with his eyes. He responded to the sound of my voice. And then, the magic happened... he smiled at me!! For the first time since I met my kid, he finally acknowledged me by giving me feedback. I can honestly tell you, as I write this, that was it. I was forever hooked on my son. We did it! We finally had a moment. I smiled at him and he smiled at me. There was a communication that had never happened before. He gave me proof that he liked me. It was the reassurance I had been waiting for. My son didn't think I was an asshole, he actually liked me! After the first smile came the extending of the arms. My son would lift his arms up and, without words, tell me, "Pick me up, Dad! I want *you* to hold me!" As I write this, my eyes are watering. I don't know why they are tearing up. In part because I almost feel guilty for not having that intense feeling of love sooner, or because I'm getting emotional because I miss that. I really miss those early days of when my son and I were exploring our relationship. It's a time in my life I will cherish forever.

Once my son and I bonded, that was it, I was addicted. Those warm fuzzy feelings I was looking so forward to feeling had *finally* arrived. He can, at a moment's notice, put a smile on my face. If I'm at work and I'm having a bad day, I pull out my phone and page through a couple pictures. It immediately puts a smile on my face. I drive home from work with this anticipation, this fuzzy feeling in my gut, not all that different to the feeling I would get Christmas morning... I can't wait to get home to see my kid.

For all those prospective dads out there, don't feel guilty. I would advise you not to expect to fall head over heels in love with your kid on day one, or even month one. The relationship with your son or daughter is no different than any other relationship in your life. You have to get to know each other first. And it's not until you get to know each other does that magic happen. Be patient. Know that fatherhood is a journey, and it's a journey we are blessed to be chosen for.

## NOBODY WILL GET IT

The more I bonded with my son, the more I wanted to climb to the highest mountain and shout to the entire world how cool my kid was, I wanted to talk to my friends and tell them when he started smiling, and I wanted to call my buddies and tell them when he started eating solid foods. Being a new parent, I quickly realized that although these events were important to me, my friends and even some family members couldn't give two shits. The reality is that friends really don't care about your kid the way you do, I mean, they'll be polite and listen to your stories, but they really don't want to hear them. A baby is always going to mean the most to his or her parents. Now, grandparents will love the kid and so will baby's aunts and uncles, but most everybody else is just being polite when you talk about your kid.

The only person I found to have the same passion about telling and listening to stories about my son and daughter was my wife. I knew if I told my wife a story about something my kids had done earlier in the day, she would listen to that story and absorb every word I said. And I would reciprocate whenever she would tell me a story. It has become a cool bond that my wife and I share.

My wife and I try to have what we call "date night." We'll drop the kids off at Grandma's house, and we'll go out to dinner. I think it's just as important to keep your marriage healthy as it is being a good parent because I believe the two go hand in hand. If you have a great marriage, it means you will stick together through thick and thin and always be together for your kids. I think kids having both a mother *and* a father might be the most important thing to them growing up. So, every now and then, my wife and I go on a date without the kids. And every time we do this, always, without a doubt, we end up smiling, laughing, and talking about our kids. Even on our one night out a year, away from our kids, we can't help but think, talk, and obsess about our kids. We both love our kids more than anything in the world. So as long as we live, we'll always have something in common.

# BUTTONS SUCK!

Okay, I'm going to paint a picture for you. It's three o'clock in the morning, and you've just been woken up by a crying baby from your deep sleep. You stumble into the kitchen, start warming a bottle, and then walk to baby's room, where you begin changing a diaper in the dark. While you're changing baby's diaper in the dark, baby is crying, pissed off, and hungry. Being pissed off, it's natural to think baby would be kicking and waving their arms all over the place, so it's obvious that you would want to complete the diaper changing process in the least amount of time possible, so baby can be quieted with a nice warm bottle. Problem is, baby is wearing pajamas with 20 buttons running from the collar all the way down to the foot and, while baby squirms around, you are trying to match up 20 tiny buttons in the dark. Nothing pissed me off more, as a parent, than having to deal with those tiny buttons in the dark. Every time my son woke up in the middle of the night and he was wearing pajamas with buttons, it would take me five minutes to button all the buttons once I was done changing the diaper. And sometimes, after the five minutes, I would have to start over again because I missed a button and my son's pajamas were now on crooked.

It's because of this disdain for buttons that I implemented a "No Button" policy in our house. My son was never allowed to go to bed wearing anything with buttons, and neither was my daughter. I hated having to deal with them. There's a simple solution to buttons: zippers. They make baby pajamas that have one zipper running from the collar all the way to the foot of the pajama. So instead of trying to button 20 tiny buttons in the pitch dark, all you have to do is zip the zipper up. It takes all but a half a second. It saves you the headache of having to deal with buttons and gets your kid to eating their bottle five minutes faster. If there is one thing that you take from this book, I want you to take this: **do not buy any pajamas with buttons!** Only buy pajamas with zippers. It will save you a ton of headaches. But good luck finding them because they are much harder to locate then the pajamas with buttons. I'm guessing it's because there are a lot of parents like me, who discovered they hate buttons, so they buy out the joint once they come across a few pairs with zippers.

# DADDERDAY

My wife is a hairstylist, and one of her busiest days of the week is Saturday. Which means, Saturday, becomes: Dadderday. It's my time to spend with my kids. I wish I could take credit for the word "Dadderday," but I first heard it from a buddy of mine. He coined the phrase because it's usually the one day a week he gets to spend with his daughter. His wife happens to work at the same salon as my wife.

It was during these "Dadderdays" that I really gained an enormous amount of respect for stay-at-home parents. One thing about babies is you can *never* ignore them. You have to constantly be at their beck and call. There is no downtime when you are watching a kid. I have no doubt in my mind that working a full-time job is way easier than being a stay-at-home parent. At least at work, I have time to screw off. If I'm bored or burnt out, I hop on the internet and bid on something, or I stroll to the toilet and take a 20-minute dump, reading sports articles on my smart phone. But when you are at home, alone watching a baby, those simple pleasures in life, like taking a dump, take a back seat to baby. If you have to take a dump and baby is hungry, baby wins. Now, this isn't so much the case in the early going. Because you can put baby in the swing and that should keep them occupied enough for you to drop a bomb or do some quick chores. But when baby starts crawling and walking, it becomes extremely difficult to do anything. You can't leave baby alone for more than 10 seconds without worrying that they are going to hurt themselves.

When my kid started walking, I implemented a little technique when I needed to go to the bathroom for an extended period of time; I would put my son in his bouncy saucer. A bouncy saucer is this thing that is in the shape of a saucer, and baby can jump up and down in it. The bouncy saucer was great when my son out grew the swing. It was a safe place we could put him in and know he was okay. But I wouldn't recommend leaving your baby unattended in that thing for very long. My friend's wife put their kid in the bouncy saucer and left him alone in the hallway while she took a shower. Well, she doesn't know how, but somehow their son had fallen over in that thing and crawled out of it. Thank God their son went in the direction of the bedroom. Because if he had gone the other way, baby probably would have tumbled down the steps. Plus, in addition to the dangers associated with leaving your baby unattended, babies hate being left alone. As babies grow up, and they become more cognizant of their surroundings, they start to hate being left alone. They always want to be by you and where the action is. I would say, starting at around five months, I could never leave the room without my son or daughter getting upset. It's kind of a double-edged sword because you can't get anything done without taking baby with you. But, the cool thing is, it makes you feel good that baby wants to be with you. I liked the fact that my kids hated when I left the room. It let me know they loved me.

Anyway, when I had to go to the bathroom and my kid was already crawling, I would put him in the bouncy saucer, and I would place the bouncy saucer right outside the bathroom door. Then I would open and close the bathroom door, playing peek-a-boo with him. For the most part, it would keep him occupied just enough for me to finish my business. Every time I would open the door, my son would smile. And then I would leave the door open, just a crack, and I would watch him trying to see me. It was a really cool way to interact with my kid. He was waiting for that moment when I opened the door. And when he

figured out that he could see me through the crack
that added another element of fun. He would look
for me and smile at me through the crack in the
door. It's those little moments that I loved. I loved
watching his brain develop, and I loved watching his
intelligence come out. At three months, baby would
never look for you through a crack in the door. But
as baby gets older and their brain starts picking up
on more and more things, you are able to play more
in-depth games.

Putting baby in the bouncy and setting him or her
outside the bathroom door also works with taking
a shower. I felt a little weird taking my kids in the
bathroom with me to shower. I wasn't sure if it was
cool being naked in front of them. I know they didn't
really know what they were seeing, but I never wanted
to see my dad naked, so I thought I would offer my
kids the same respect. Anyway, to take a shower I put
my kids in the bouncy, and I kept the bathroom door
open. Then I would play peek-a-boo with the shower
curtain. Every time, without fail, my kids would smile
when I said "peek-a-boo!" Then I would mess with
them and pop my head out from different ends of
the bathtub. That really got them going because they
never knew if I was going to peek out of the back of

the tub or the front of the tub.

Basically, when you are home alone with the baby, you have to be creative. You have to do whatever you need to do to get the job done. In order for me to wash dishes after breakfast, I would put my son in his high chair and I would sing, jump around, and make goofy sounds. My neighbors probably thought I was nuts, but it was the only thing that would keep my kid happy enough to sit in his highchair long enough for me to wash the dishes. Usually, the second my son was done eating, he wanted out. And if I didn't keep him entertained, he was sure to let me know.

I really looked forward to my Dadderdays, but they were exhausting. By the time my wife got home, which was about three o'clock on Saturdays, my son had usually kicked my ass. He was non-stop with wanting to be entertained and wanting a new change of environment every 30 minutes. I don't know if all babies are like this around five months, but when my kid hit five months, he couldn't sit still. He constantly had to be on the move. If we were in the living room, he could only stay there for a few minutes before he was bored and wanted to cruise off into another room. I learned the best way to occupy my kid was to give him anything that wasn't dangerous and wasn't a toy. I would give him a measuring cup and he would think it was the coolest thing in the world. My son would look at it with such amazement, almost like he was marveling at the genius idea of putting lines with numbers on the side of a cup.

## Empower Yourself

As I'm winding down this book, I hope there is at least a nugget or two of information that will help you as you prepare to become a parent. I tried to be as open and honest with my feelings as possible in an effort to give you a peek into one man's mind as I made the transition into parenthood. I can say that this has been a bit of a therapeutic experience for me. I started writing this book rather quickly after my son was born, and then put the book down. Then, several years later, after my daughter was born, I picked the book back up and read through it. I can say that in reading it a few years later, I'm glad from a personal standpoint that I did it. I had forgotten stuff that I'd written years before, so I'm very happy for no other reason than that it almost turned into a diary of sorts that helped me shine a light on memories that had faded while living each new day with my family.

I had my wife read this book, and I asked her if she thought there was anything in here that might help people. She told me that she hoped people would take away one important thing. My wife wants this book to _empower_ you as new parents. She hopes that you realize that although doctors and nurses are in a position of authority and have more medical knowledge, it doesn't give them the right to push you around as new parents into how "they" want the birth of your child to go. The birthing process is an extremely intimate and primal experience that, as the parents, you retain 100% control over. If you, as parents, don't want to have the doctors intervene, it is your right to not have a medical intervention. If you want to delay the chord cutting or opt out of giving your child a Hepatitis vaccine in their first seconds of life, you have the right to do that. If you don't want to bombard your fetus in the early stages of development with ultrasound waves, opt out of getting an ultrasound in your first few doctor visits. Conversely, if the stress of giving birth is bringing unbearable anxiety, it's your right as a parent to take medication that takes the edge off, and if you can't wait to see your baby once you realize your pregnant, then get the ultrasound. I don't believe there is any one perfect way to give birth. At the end of the day, all that really matters is that your child is born into this world healthy. My son's birthing day and my daughter's birthing day were two completely different experiences but, again, all that really matters is that they both came into this world healthy.

I always knew I wanted to become a parent. I just never really knew when the perfect time was for me. It's not until becoming a parent that I realized the answer to that question. *Anytime* is the perfect time to become a parent. I believe everyone in the world should feel the love between a parent and a child. It's a love so strong and so pure that nothing in the world compares to it, and I hope and pray that every person reading this book is blessed with a perfectly healthy child. I wish you nothing but the absolute best in your transition into parenthood. Please, every so often, take a beat to absorb everything. Relish the late nights staying up with your baby, embrace the days when they are small enough to sleep on your shoulders, and welcome all the stages that come with a child growing up. Although becoming a parent is permanent, your child's youth is not. There will be a day when they grow up, leave our nests and, hopefully, start their own family. They say that the future of the world is in the hands of our youth. I don't believe that. I believe the future of the world rests in the hands of *us* parents. It's our duty as the parents to teach our kids the proper way to live. To treat all people with respect, embrace each other's differences, and accept everyone for who they are. If every parent in the world did that, I think we might end up leaving this world a better place than when we found it.